AF262884

Estrogen,
Interrupted

Estrogen, Interrupted

A GUIDE TO SURVIVING AND THRIVING IN PERIMENOPAUSE

Rebecca Dunsmoor-Su, MD, and
Amy Voedisch, MD

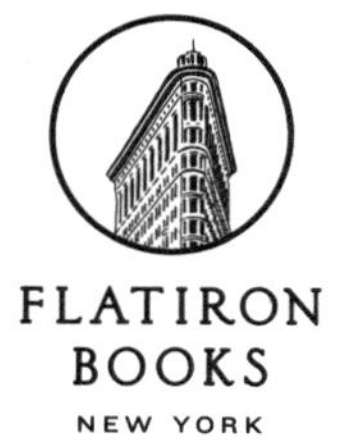

FLATIRON
BOOKS
NEW YORK

ESTROGEN, INTERRUPTED. Copyright © 2026 by Rebecca Dunsmoor-Su and Amy Voedisch. All rights reserved. Printed in the United States of America. For information, address Flatiron Books, 120 Broadway, New York, NY 10271. EU Representative: Macmillan Publishers Ireland Ltd., 1st Floor, The Liffey Trust Centre, 117–126 Sheriff Street Upper, Dublin 1, D01 YC43.

www.flatironbooks.com

The Library of Congress Cataloging-in-Publication Data is available upon request.

ISBN 978-1-250-38980-0 (hardcover)
ISBN 978-1-250-38981-7 (ebook)

Our books may be purchased in bulk for specialty retail/wholesale, literacy, corporate/premium, educational, and subscription box use. Please contact MacmillanSpecialMarkets@macmillan.com.

First Edition: 2026

10 9 8 7 6 5 4 3 2 1

Contents

Introduction: We Believe Women   1

PART ONE
YOUR NEW "NORMAL"

1   Are You in Perimenopause? And What Exactly Is It Anyway?   11

2   The Hormonal Life Cycle: From First Period to Last and Everything In Between   27

PART TWO
ALL CHANGES, GREAT AND SMALL

3   Erratic Periods: Coping with the Ebbs and Flows   41

4   Bad Night's Sleep: The Curse of the 2 A.M. Wake-Up Call   55

5   Mood Swings: Like PMS on Steroids   71

6   Vagina Trouble: Dryness and Other Discomforts   89

7   Disappearing Libido: Not Tonight, I Have Perimenopause   101

8   Swelling Waistline: The Midlife Middle   115

9   Brain Fog: A Disorganized Mind   133

10   Skin and Hair Woes: Women Take It on the Chin   143

11   Hot Flashes and Night Sweats: Swelter Skelter   157

PART THREE
COMPREHENSIVE TREATMENTS

12   Contraception. Yep, Contraception! Why You Might Need It Now   171

13   Menopausal Hormone Therapy: Resurrecting a Reputation   187

14   Everything Else: Nonhormonal Treatments   199

PART FOUR
NEXT STEPS: MENOPAUSE AND LIFELONG WELLNESS

15   Cardiovascular Health: Your Heart Needs Love and Attention   209

16   Breast Cancer: What You Can Do to Protect Yourself   219

17   Bone Density: Now Is the Time to Prevent Breaks Later   232

   Coda: Talking to Your Doctor, Being Heard, and Taking Control of Your Well-Being   243

Acknowledgments   253

References   255

Index   271

Estrogen, Interrupted

Introduction

Not-so-funny story: Woman walks into a doctor's office and says, "I'm really having a hard time sleeping—I get so hot it wakes me up nightly—and I feel very on edge, angry one day, sad and on the verge of tears the next. I'll walk into a room and not remember what I came in for and please don't ask me to dredge up the name of that actress in the movie I just saw, or the author of the book I read last month. I'm still exercising and I swear I'm avoiding sugar, but my pants don't fit. I didn't get my period for months and I thought I was pregnant (how, I can't explain because I never feel like having sex!). Next thing I know, I'm bleeding so much it's like a scene from a horror movie. Doctor, what's wrong with me?"

"It's normal," he says. "Eat healthy!"

An enraging response, but, sadly, it's not an uncommon one. The symptoms, the silence, and the lack of understanding of perimenopause all play out against a backdrop of medicine's long history of shrugging off women's concerns. No doubt the misogyny dates back to time immemorial, but we have the ancient Greeks to thank for the term "hysteria," derived from the Greek word for uterus (*hystera*) and applied to women's "problems" for centuries. And so it is that even in this day and age, something that happens exclusively to women—perimenopause— elicits hardly an eye blink from many doctors. How many of us have heard "she's just hysterical" used to brush off a woman's very real concerns?

But, of course, you're not hysterical. Crazy things may be happening, but *you're* not crazy. When you say that you don't feel like yourself, that you're bewildered, uncomfortable, perhaps even suffering, we believe you. We've been there ourselves and we've seen hundreds of patients in the same boat. Not only do you have a right to be taken seriously; you have a right to know how to manage your symptoms so you can feel better. And there's a proven path to doing just that.

Sometimes it may seem that the days when women's health conditions were ignored are long past. After all, in recent years, advertisers have boldly marketed products to menopausal women. Actresses have appeared in the media to share their personal experience with brain fog and scaly skin. When *The New York Times Magazine* published the article "Women Have Been Misled About Menopause" by Susan Dominus, it went viral.

We couldn't be more thrilled that after years of dismissal by both the medical community and society at large, menopause is finally getting some of the attention it deserves. *But perimenopause is not menopause!* Menopause is the complete cessation of your periods. If you haven't had your period for twelve months, you're in menopause. Perimenopause ("around menopause") is less clearly defined. You still get your period, but your reproductive system is in flux, and that can cause system-wide disruption. In fact, while menopause may get all the press, the symptoms of perimenopause can be even more pronounced than those of menopause. Nonetheless, in the course of trying to explain what they're going through, many perimenopausal women are met with blank stares and even condescension—*You're still young, you're still getting your period, you're not in menopause, don't worry about it!* One of our favorites was reported by a patient whose (male) primary care physician told her, "Women have done this for thousands of years. It's not a big deal. You don't need to do anything about it."

Their message: Stop talking. Our message: Start talking more. There's no need to suffer in silence. Perimenopause is challenging and it can last a long time. It's a marathon, not a sprint, and the symptoms can be very distressing, especially if it takes you by surprise. It's quite likely that no one mentioned that, about the time you're in your late thirties, maybe early forties (though it can even begin in your early thirties), you may start waking up in the middle of the night, every night, and your periods may sometimes become very heavy, sometimes very light, and sometimes very irregular. Your hairline may change and your skin become drier, and you may begin gaining weight. You may have brain fog or low libido. You may get depressed, anxious, and so irritable that it impacts your relationships.

There's no shortage of books and other resources available to prepare us for pregnancy. And just about every fifth-grade girl learns what to expect when her period arrives, or at least she's urged to read *Are You There God? It's Me, Margaret*. Why aren't women in their thirties and forties given a similar manual about what perimenopause will bring? Where are the soothing Judy Blume stories for grownups?

Women deserve to be apprised of every phase of their reproductive lives and informed about all the treatment options available to them. In this book, we're going to share everything about the perimenopausal body so that, armed with good information, you can better advocate for yourself if and when you seek care. And we do urge you to seek care if your symptoms are negatively impacting your life. There's no reason to be stoic. Just because your neighbor down the street never had a hot flash or your partner doesn't understand why you need to lower the thermostat at night doesn't mean that your symptoms aren't real and that they don't warrant treatment. If there's one thing that we've learned over our years of practice, it's that there is not one blueprint for the way perimenopause will play out. There are so many varied symptoms—some that you might never even associate with your reproductive system, like joint pain—and every single person is going to have a different combination of those symptoms and to varying degrees. Perimenopause's unpredictability is predictable—it's a wild ride.

We're here to offer guidance as you go through this sometimes long, often strange trip through midlife. The menopausal transition—a collective term for all the stages up to your final menstrual period (FMP)—is our area of expertise, the focus of both our practices, and a subject we've published articles about in medical literature. We go to conferences, read the research, and most importantly, we listen, then we listen some more. Just about every single day, women tell us what they're going through, and because we've immersed ourselves in this area of medicine and learned so much from working with perimenopausal patients, we've got answers for them—and for you.

But it wasn't always so. Most people don't know that obstetricians and gynecologists (ob-gyns), presumably knowledgeable about all things relating to the reproductive system, don't receive robust training in perimenopausal and menopausal medicine. In medical school, perimenopause and menopause are barely mentioned, and in residency (after we finish medical school, we enter residency to learn our specialties), we have four years to learn every possible complication of pregnancy and delivery as well as how to do complex gynecologic surgeries. There's not a lot of time left over to acquire knowledge about the care of women going through the menopausal transition. Doctors who train in primary care have similar limitations; they have three years to study general medicine and rarely have the opportunity to learn much about perimenopause and menopause. Our experience training to be ob-gyns followed the usual pattern, but later in our careers we both were hit with what felt like a lightning bolt: Women in midlife were crying out for help, and we were going to answer the call.

That said, we found our path to this calling in different ways. Rebecca went to medical school at the University of Pennsylvania, where she received her MD and a master's in clinical epidemiology. She did her residency at the University of Pennsylvania hospital before moving to Seattle and spending years practicing as an ob-gyn, serving on the faculty of the University of Washington. Then came a couple of "aha" moments. In 2002, a press release announced that a large study called the Women's Health Initiative (WHI), which was testing hormone replacement therapy in menopausal women, was abruptly ended because of a perceived breast cancer risk to the study's participants. (We'll talk more about this study in chapter 15.) It instigated a wave of panic and left many menopausal women perplexed about how best to manage their symptoms. Once the publication and data were released, Rebecca and her colleagues could tell right away that the study's results had been misinterpreted, as they were later proven to be. Seeing so many women miserable after the WHI study press release was Rebecca's "aha" moment number one—these were patients who needed guidance.

The second stroke of inspiration came when, in the wake of the vilification of hormone therapy, a wave of practitioners (many of them not doctors) began offering perimenopausal and menopausal women "safe and effective" remedies that were either not actually safe or not actually effective (or both). It was infuriating. Having done a lot of reproductive endocrinology training as a resident, Rebecca was slightly ahead of the curve when she came face-to-face with patients in the menopausal transition. But she could also see that the research and theories presented to doctors through journals and conferences didn't translate into practical knowledge of how to help women facing difficult midlife symptoms. In 2019, she founded a menopause-focused practice at Swedish Medical Center in Seattle and never looked back. She's now the chief medical officer of a large national telemedicine company for perimenopause and menopause.

Amy went to medical school at Mayo Clinic in Minnesota and moved to the Bay Area in California for ob-gyn residency. She then further trained in complex family planning at Stanford University, meanwhile earning a master's in clinical sciences research. From there she focused on increasing access to contraception in underserved international areas, and maintained a clinical practice at Stanford. In the course of working at one of Stanford's suburban clinics, Amy unexpectedly found herself inundated with patients over the age of forty, who had a lot of questions about perimenopause—questions she couldn't answer. So she worked on extending her knowledge and became a Menopause Society Certified Practitioner (we both are) and loves it (we both do).

And then we met. On a Facebook group for ob-gyn moms. Over the course of our conversations, we discovered we both felt that our perimenopausal patients were underserved. Perimenopause, we agreed, is also a collective problem, an issue in need of much greater research and attention. And wouldn't it be great, we thought, if more women understood why they're undergoing so many changes at this time of life? If more women could go to their doctors equipped with the right information so they know what questions to ask? If more women knew what all their treatment options are?

If it sounds like we're on a mission, well, we are. We want perimenopause to get the menopause treatment—that is, to be something women now talk openly about, that physicians are well-versed in, and that society at large (particularly partners of perimenopausal women) acknowledges is a natural, if potentially tough time that women may need some help with. In the meantime, everything we know right now about how to address perimenopausal symptoms awaits you in the pages of this book. Our approach to helping women feel better is informed by science. Although we're great believers in trying things that may help as long as they don't hurt, we're also strong proponents of going where the evidence leads. Both of us have had many, many patients come through the door who've spent money on "cures" that, at best, don't deliver, and at worst put their health in real danger. We want to help you make informed, safe choices that fit with both your personal viewpoint and your unique body. And we've got nothing to sell. We're not going to ask you to buy our supplements or a batch of herbs. We simply have a lot of information and we want to share what we know.

So, what you'll find on the pages ahead: A thorough examination of perimenopausal symptoms—we've heard them all, the big, the little, the quirky, the embarrassing. We discuss, dissect, and demystify the role hormonal ups and downs *and* life's ups and downs (including the inevitable process of aging) play in symptoms you may encounter. We'll talk, too, about your options for reducing symptom severity and, in some cases, making some symptoms go away altogether. And we'll cover what you need to know going forward: The menopausal transition can raise the likelihood of several health conditions, including osteoporosis and heart disease. The last chapters of this book will describe how to minimize the risks and optimize the postmenopausal stage of your life.

These are all issues we cover with our patients during office hours. You, on the contrary, may be reading this far from our Palo Alto and Seattle practices, perhaps tucked into bed before turning out the lights at night (or maybe in lieu of staring at the ceiling at 2 a.m.—you are perimenopausal after all). Whenever, wherever, by the time you turn the last page of this book, we hope it feels like you've just had a long session with the doctor of your dreams: Someone who gets what you're going through—and knows how to help.

Part One

Your New "Normal"

1

Are You in Perimenopause?

And What Exactly Is It Anyway?

I feel like I'm at war with my body.

—FORTY-FIVE-YEAR-OLD PERIMENOPAUSAL PATIENT

It was a long meeting, but Heather was used to that. She'd been working for the data systems company for ten years and she was regularly outspoken at those lengthy business gatherings, throwing out ideas and amusing her colleagues with her signature witty repartee. Heather is smart and funny, a wisecracker by nature, but on this particular day she was finding it hard to stay engaged and follow along with the discussion. Though she was usually very confident, she felt insecure and anxious. Part of it was that her thinking felt fuzzy; part of it was that she was terrified she was going to have a hot flash and end up in an embarrassing pool of sweat. This was a scenario that would play out again and again in the months to come.

"Something was happening to me, and I didn't know what it was," she says. "It was like I was in a new body. I even smelled different to myself. And it wasn't a slow change. It seemed to happen all of a sudden."

Once a ballet dancer, Heather barely recognized herself when she looked down at a now fleshy waistline. She was waking up several times during the night and had started having panic attacks in the shower. "In the shower? Why? I couldn't explain it. And neither could my doctor. I just wanted someone to tell me, 'Here's what you're going through and here's what will happen next.'"

If you've picked up this book, you might have had a diagnosis of perimenopause, or you might just have a hunch that, based on your symptoms, you've hit that midlife milestone. How can you know for sure? Contrary to what many practitioners might suggest, there's no simple test that provides the answer. (Well, there are tests, but unreliable ones, and in most cases we don't use them, for reasons we'll explain shortly.)

The defining factor of perimenopause is that it's a time when your body's production of the hormones estrogen and progesterone begins to drop precipitously as the march toward menopause commences. But these hormones, known as sex or reproductive hormones, do not descend in a gradual straight line. Nor is the transition like a skier gently descending a bunny hill. Instead, perimenopause is characterized by dramatic ups and downs. One month your hormones are at the top of a steep black diamond run, the next month they're down at the lodge sipping hot cocoa. Then they ride the gondola back up to the top again only to make another descent. These ups and downs are what may leave you feeling alternately fine and completely alien to yourself. Your hormone levels can change from day to day, normal to irregular, high to low. This explains, at least partly, why the symptoms of perimenopause can be so dramatic, and confusing—and why it can be hard to diagnose.

Hormone-level tests do exist, but the hormonal variability occurring during this time of life tends to make them a waste of time and money. Even in the throes of perimenopause, it's entirely likely that any hormone testing may catch you on a day when your hormones happen to be behaving normally, making it impossible for the screening to provide a definitive answer as to whether you've hit perimenopause.

Which brings us to the question: How *do* you know? The way we diagnose perimenopause is based on the symptoms, all of which you'll read about in the upcoming chapters. If you're experiencing one or more of them, and you're in the perimenopausal age bracket, you're very likely in perimenopause. And that's good to know; it will explain a lot and, hopefully, calm any fears you have that something is very wrong with you.

But "perimenopause," the descriptor for what's happening, is really just a jumping-off point. Ultimately what you and your health practitioner will want to do is address your symptoms one by one. That's what this book is intended to help you do. But first, we'll peek beneath the hood. What, anatomically speaking, is perimenopause? What causes this state of metamorphosis? As unsettling as it all can be, the hormone-driven ups and downs of perimenopause are completely normal. We'll get to all that in chapter 2. But first we want to talk about some general aspects of perimenopause, as well as how other facets of midlife may influence your experience.

Where Perimenopause Falls in the Grand Scheme of Things

Perimenopause is part of a continuum of stages the female reproductive system goes through during the course of one's life. The following terms describe the stopping points along that continuum, each having to do with the ovaries, the eggs they produce, and the hormones that keep the whole show running. While you may feel the effects of each stage in all areas of your body, from your head down to your toenails, it all begins with signals from the brain that affect the uterus and ovaries. Bear in mind as you read through these definitions that they describe what *typically* happens during each phase. Your individual experience may vary, and that's perfectly normal.

<u>Puberty</u>: At this stage, the brain prompts hormonal changes that spur physical developments (breasts, pubic and other body hair) and set in motion the process that will allow you to conceive. Getting your period is a sign that your reproductive system is producing viable (i.e., fertilizable) eggs. Most girls go through puberty and get their first period anywhere from age nine to age thirteen.

<u>Premenopause</u>: This is the (usually) decades-long phase between your first period and the beginning of perimenopause. Your body is steadily producing estrogen and progesterone, the two major hormones that regulate your reproductive cycle (and influence many other functions). The eggs in your ovaries are of good quality and you're ovulating at a more or less regular clip, usually about every twenty-eight days.

<u>Perimenopause</u>: This is the reproductive chapter that falls in between the relatively smooth-going premenopause phase and menopause, which is defined as the stage of life when your periods cease altogether. It doesn't have a specific start date; perimenopause typically begins when you're in your early forties, but it can begin as early as around age thirty-five or as late as your fifties. It can last a few years but can also last a decade.

The most "scientific" way to describe what happens during perimenopause is to say that everything goes bananas. In perimenopause, a dwindling supply of viable eggs causes your hormones to bounce up and down. This may cause you to have erratic periods, but that's not always a sign of perimenopause. Many people, including some healthcare providers, think that having normal, predictable periods cancels out a diagnosis of perimenopause, but that's not the case.

Rebecca had a patient just the other day who said, "I'm thirty-eight and I feel like things are changing. I'm moody. I have more anxiety. Sex is a little painful now and it never was before. I have chin hair! But my periods are still pretty regular. I've seen three doctors who've all said, 'Nope, it can't be perimenopause.'" Sure it can. It doesn't matter if your cycle is still regular. If you feel something is changing, and it's been determined that nothing else is wrong, let's call it perimenopause. The upshot is that there's no one marker, no one neon sign pointing to your uterus and flashing "perimenopause." There are lots of different symptoms, and you may have some, but not others. Every woman's experience of perimenopause is unique.

<u>Menopause</u>: The average age of the onset of menopause is fifty-one (the range of "normal" ages is forty-five to fifty-five). Unlike perimenopause, menopause does have a definitive start date that lets you identify when it's arrived: Once you've gone a full year without a period, you are in menopause. ("In menopause" and "postmenopausal" are the same thing, and the terms are often used interchangeably.) Occasionally, someone will reach that marker, then a few months later have a period. Whether you start the clock over at this point or not doesn't really matter, because the lack of bleeding for so many months means that the main determinant of menopause—your ovaries are no longer developing eggs for potential fertilization or producing much estrogen and progesterone—is well underway.

<u>Surgical Menopause</u>: When both ovaries are removed for a medical reason, such as endometriosis or to reduce the risk of ovarian cancer, you automatically enter menopause, no matter your age. Rebecca has firsthand experience with surgical menopause, but more about that later.

HORMONAL CONDITIONS THAT AFFECT PERIMENOPAUSE

There are two conditions we want to discuss that can affect the age of perimenopausal onset and exacerbate certain symptoms. If you have either of these, you're likely already talking to your physician about how they might impact your experience of the menopausal transition, but we want to make sure to flag them here since they can impact the kinds of treatments you consider and your broader timeline.

POLYCYSTIC OVARY SYNDROME (PCOS)

Between 7 to 10 percent of women in their childbearing years have PCOS, and the signs—irregular periods, facial hair, acne, weight gain around the middle—can be very similar to those of perimenopause. Some of the PCOS symptoms arise for the same reasons they do in perimenopause: Many follicles work hard to develop eggs, but those eggs rarely make it to ovulation. So, as with people in perimenopause, women with PCOS can have irregular and sometimes very heavy periods.

But there's an important difference between PCOS and perimenopause. In perimenopause, the eggs have aged; their poor quality is at the root of the failure to ovulate. With PCOS, for reasons we don't quite understand (but may have something to do with insulin resistance), the follicles make different patterns of hormones, which impedes the development of the eggs. There's nothing wrong with the eggs; they're just not getting the assistance they need to grow. Another thing that goes wrong is that cells inside the ovaries produce excessive amounts of testosterone and other male sex hormones (androgens). This also hinders ovulation, and is mostly to blame for the errant hairs, pimples, and belly fat that can be symptoms of PCOS.

Girls can develop PCOS as early as when they first start menstruating, though it's more likely to become apparent when a woman is in her twenties or thirties. Birth control pills do a good job of helping stabilize the menstrual cycle and fixing some of the hormonal imbalances of PCOS, but because people with PCOS produce and use insulin differently than other people, we treat them a lot like we treat diabetics. Some are prescribed metformin, a common type 2 diabetes drug, and we encourage PCOS patients to lose weight and manage their carbohydrate intake.

If you have PCOS, reaching perimenopause can be like a double whammy, exacerbating an already unreliable chain of reproductive events. Your brain, already fighting to get an egg to ovulation because of the PCOS, now has to fight even harder to make ovulation happen. That *may* ramp up the perimenopausal symptoms for some (though not all) women with PCOS. PCOS may also delay the onset of menopause, with some studies showing that the FMP may come one to two years later than the average age of menopause.

PREMATURE OVARIAN INSUFFICIENCY (POI)

Premature ovarian insufficiency is a condition that occurs when the ovaries more or less shut down before the normal age of menopause. In women with POI, early perimenopausal symptoms like irregular periods can occur when they're in their teens, twenties, or thirties, before and sometimes long before the usual age of transition. It may then quickly lead to the complete cessation of periods—menopause.

POI affects 1 to 2 percent of women under the age of forty, and only about .01 percent under the age of thirty. We don't really know why some women develop POI. It can be a genetic anomaly, and some research suggests the ovaries' premature depletion is related to auto-immune conditions and even influenced by environmental factors. POI is often referred to as early menopause, but that's a misnomer. Early menopause occurs between the ages of forty and forty-five (again, the median age of menopause onset is fifty-one); POI comes even earlier. For that reason—and because the abrupt and steep dip in estrogen at such a young age can pose a serious threat to both cardiac health and bone health—we generally treat it aggressively with hormone therapy. The hormones aren't to treat the symptoms per se, though there will be relief. More significantly, they're there to protect your heart, your brain, and your bones from estrogen loss. If you're under forty and experiencing perimenopausal or menopausal symptoms, it's very important to see your physician for a full workup.

Who Experiences the Menopausal Transition—and Why?

One of the interesting things about the perimenopause and menopause phases of the reproductive continuum is that they are an almost uniquely human affliction. There are a few other species that scientists have determined also cease to produce eggs after a certain age. One is a specific group of chimpanzees called the Ngogo that live in Uganda; the other species are five types of whales: killer, false killer, beluga, short fin, and narwhals. But the majority of mammals do not experience menopause, meaning they can theoretically reproduce up until death. No one knows for sure why female mammals, including female humans, have evolved to experience menopause, but there are a few theories, most revolving around the idea that it may give a species an evolutionary edge.

For instance, when an older female whale can no longer become pregnant, it ensures that she and her offspring will not be competing for resources with her daughter's offspring. This increases the likelihood of survival within the group. Another possible explanation is the "grandmother hypothesis," which posits that females not busy with their own children can help with their grandchildren, again increasing the likelihood that the genes they passed down will have a greater chance of survival. (Also part of the grandmother theory is the idea that these older "women" have accumulated such a wealth of valuable knowledge that it doesn't make sense to lose them, and pregnancy is riskier as one gets older.) If either of these theories is correct, it may explain what nature had in mind when creating the menopausal transition (but why did it have to include hot flashes? Why? Why? We don't know)—even if these theories don't relate to how we live our lives today.

In our human world, the menopausal transition is exclusive to people with a female reproductive system. (The phrases "male menopause" or "andropause" get thrown around a lot and may be a metaphor for some type of midlife crisis, but they are not tied to any significant changes in the male hormones and reproductive system.) While we recognize that there are a number of people who experience menopause and don't identify as women, most of the research we'll talk about has been done on cis women.

If you're a trans woman, you won't naturally go through perimenopause or menopause, but if you want to—and some trans women do— your doctor can help you adjust your estrogen medication (if you're taking it) to make it possible. If you're a trans man, the advancing menopausal transition can be fraught. The good news for trans men anxious about the possibility of hormonal changes taking them back to a gendered experience is that supplemental testosterone will prevent ovaries from functioning in a way that leads to the traditional menopausal pathway. They will function somewhat, though, and that is a positive thing, as the small amount of estrogen they produce helps protect bone and cardiovascular health.

It's important that everyone who experiences perimenopause is included in the conversation, just as it's important that the conversation be meaningful and ongoing. And there have been some hopeful signs that progress is being made in that area. One of the high points came in 2023 when lawmakers introduced the Menopause Research and Equity Act, which required the director of the National Institutes of Health (NIH) to evaluate the results and status of completed and ongoing research related to menopause and perimenopause. It also mandated that the NIH conduct and support additional research. The legislation has not been passed yet and time will tell if the legislation was a one-off or a sign of continuing progress in women's health research. We are, of course, hoping that it's the latter.

ENVIRONMENTAL FACTORS

We live in a dirty world, with chemicals and plastics infiltrating everything from cosmetics, furniture, carpets, and cleaning and building materials to clothing, food packaging, and food itself. Then they infiltrate us. "Microplastics have been found in every single organ in the human body," reports Jane van Dis, MD, assistant professor of obstetrics and gynecology at the University of Rochester and co-founder of OBGYNs for a Sustainable Future. "So have forever chemicals, also known as PFAS (per- and polyfluoroalkyl substances) which make things non-stick and resistant to water."

While we know that toxic chemicals are all over the world, there is still a lot to be learned about how they impact the body. But research has provided some insight and, in particular, shone a light on how they affect hormones and, by extension, the menopausal transition. Many toxic chemicals are what's known as endocrine disruptors. They interfere with the endocrine (hormonal) system by binding to receptors, preventing hormones from delivering the messages they're meant to transmit. Investigators have found four primary ways hormonal disruption has the potential to impact how you experience perimenopause and menopause:

1. <u>Earlier menopausal transition</u>. A look at data from the National Health and Nutrition Examination Survey (NHANES) from 1999 to 2008, which included 31,575 menopausal women, found that the women who had the highest level of phthalates in their urine began menopause 3.17–3.8 years earlier than women with lower levels.

2. <u>An increase in the number and severity of hot flashes</u>. The NHANES data also showed that women with more phthalates in their system had a greater likelihood of hot flashes as well as more frequent flashes.

3. <u>Faster egg depletion</u>. The culprit here is bisphenol A (BPA). Found in eyeglasses, water bottles, some water supply pipes, and in the lining of metal cans (although, after warnings, most of it has now been replaced by other chemicals—which have their own hazards), BPA has been associated with low fertility. This has the potential to lead to more of the hormonal ups and downs we'll describe in chapter 2.

4. <u>Alterations in sex hormone levels</u>. Chemicals can change the pattern of estrogen, progesterone, and testosterone secretion. How this plays out in perimenopause and menopause is uncertain, but it could have something to do with the earlier onset of the transition.

While no one escapes exposure to chemicals, the degree of exposure and how deeply it affects your experience of perimenopause may depend on the environment right outside your door. If, for instance, you live in an area where the air and water quality is poor and you're close to, say, heavily fertilized farmland or industrial waste, you have a higher likelihood of struggling with symptoms. How can you address these issues? Because they're so pervasive, it's not easy to lower your exposure to chemicals. But being more mindful of what you buy and what you consume can go a long way toward helping you avoid contact with toxins.

Beyond Hormones

While perimenopause and menopause symptoms are mostly related to changes in hormones, particularly estrogen levels, hormones can't be blamed for everything. (They're also not the cure for everything, which we'll get to later.) Midlife is a phase when aging, lifestyle choices, life circumstances, and, yes, hormonal shifts all collide. As noted earlier, environmental factors can also play a role. While some symptoms, like erratic periods, for instance, are firmly rooted in hormonal changes, most are the result of a number of instigators.

Perimenopause doesn't exist in a vacuum. As you begin to consider what treatments you might want to discuss with your doctor, and what solutions you might pursue on your own, consider the big picture of midlife. A raft of different factors can contribute to the changes you're experiencing, but the three most significant beyond hormones are aging, the sometimes-insanity of everyday life, and the uniqueness of your own body.

Aging

In a sense, the menopausal transition *is* aging; it's aging of the reproductive system. But, of course, that's not the only part of your body that ages. Genetics is instrumental to how well we age, but even those who've won the genetic lottery can lose some of that good fortune if they haven't been attentive to their health or circumstances have been working against them (say, living in a very polluted area, or experiencing trauma). This can especially become apparent in midlife, a time when we bump up against many of the health-related decisions we made in our twenties and thirties.

It would be nice if we could construct a chart and place the heading "attributable to general aging" in one column and the heading "attributable to perimenopause" in another. Unfortunately, the human body doesn't quite work that way. But sometimes we can parse out some differences between the two. For instance, sleep disturbances are often due to an amalgam of factors. But certain aspects of sleeplessness are more linked to age than to changes in estrogen.

For instance, for both men and women, sleep patterns change as the years advance—although the patterns change more dramatically for women. We tend to put all sleep problems in one big bucket, but there are in fact many different aspects to poor sleep. Take sleep duration—the total amount of time you sleep per night—which declines with each passing decade. The different phases of sleep also change with age, so, while the effects of poorer sleep may become more noticeable during perimenopause, they're not necessarily *caused* by perimenopause. What *is* usually attributable to perimenopause is the exhausting cycle of waking up after you've fallen asleep, something sleep researchers call "waking after sleep onset" (WASO). That's the type of sleep problem we more commonly see with shifting estrogen levels and is associated with menopausal-related modifications in brain chemistry. (More on sleep in chapter 5.)

Weight gain is another slippery symptom. We know that estrogen loss is instrumental in not only gaining weight but also where that weight is distributed (in the middle of the body). But another cause of weight gain—a slowing metabolism—is attributable to system-wide aging. As we grow older, we lose muscle, the most calorie-hungry tissue in the body, and that drives down our metabolism—the rate at which our body burns energy.

Aging is also associated with mental changes. If you've ever spent time with people in their elder years, you know that it's not just women who suffer from memory loss. Both men's and women's brains show signs of age. Even as early as in your forties, your brain can begin to lose some of its plasticity; that is, its ability to adapt to change and create new connections. Less plasticity inhibits not only your memory but your ability to learn, too. Over the years, the brain can also become subject to microinsults as age creates changes in the blood vessels, changes that include a buildup of plaque as well as less flexibility and plasticity in the walls of the blood vessels themselves. This can contribute to neurodegenerative decline and diseases such as dementia and Alzheimer's. That said, not all memory issues during this time are strictly age-related. Women experience specific changes related to the menopausal transition. In fact, new research suggests that there are more changes in the brain during perimenopause and menopause than previously known. If you're finding your thinking is muddled, your focus is off, and your forgetfulness rising, you can likely attribute these symptoms to perimenopause, possibly combined with the many demands on your time and energy during this time.

Everyday Stressors

For so many women, "juggling" is embedded in their daily reality—something else to consider as you assess what you're going through right now. When patients come to us with a range of physiological symptoms, we often ask them to step back and tell us how their lives are going more generally. Midlife can be very busy, with everything from kids, work, aging parents, financial responsibility, and more tugging at you. Sometimes it's like when you have fifteen windows open on your computer, and you get the color ball going around and around and around—essentially your computer telling you it's on overload. If you, too, are on overload, you may experience certain symptoms associated with perimenopause—particularly those related to your mental health like anxiety, depression, moodiness, and irritability—or feel them more strongly.

For instance, when Heather was struggling with her array of typical perimenopausal symptoms, including those panic attacks in the shower, she was also still coping with the sudden death of her ex-husband and its effects on their teenage son. The incident had passed, but the trauma and grief hadn't. While, in hindsight, she can see the association between the severity of some of her symptoms, Heather didn't make the connection at the time because she was simultaneously experiencing so many other hormone-driven symptoms. Whatever the cause, it was important for her to get help, but how the problem was addressed might have depended on its origins. It's the same for all symptoms: Looking at the problem from all angles will yield the most effective solutions.

The Uniqueness of You

There's a basic blueprint for how the reproductive cycle operates, the details of which you'll read about in the next chapter. But there's also variability among individual women. It's important to be aware that everyone's body "reads" hormones differently and responds to those hormones in a particular way. There's a constellation of symptoms that can emerge during perimenopause, and because you're a unique being, you may experience some, none, or all of them. Some women breeze through the transition; some women are hit really hard.

The timing of perimenopause and menopause can vary, too. From global studies, we've learned that women in Africa, Latin America, the Middle East, and Asia tend to start the transition at a younger age than women in Europe, Australia, and the United States. Within the United States, Black women start menopause about 1.2 years earlier than white women, according to 2023 research from the SWAN study. (SWAN stands for the Study of Women's Health Across the Nation and refers to an ongoing, multisite, and multiethnic study that began in 1994 and has involved over three thousand women.) One of the SWAN investigations, this one from 2009 and published by researchers at the Albert Einstein College of Medicine in New York, also found that Black and Hispanic women had higher rates of both premature (before age forty) and early (between the ages of forty and forty-five) menopause than white and Asian women.

There may be many reasons for the disparities, some plainer than others. For instance, Black women have higher rates of fibroids (noncancerous growths in the uterus), which may be why they have a greater incidence of hysterectomy in general, and some proportion of those women will have their ovaries removed as well, putting them into surgical menopause. Black women also tend to have more intense symptoms during the menopausal transition. Again, there may be a genetic factor, but it's also abundantly clear that the stress of racism in our society plus racial bias in medicine can have an impact on how women of color experience the menopausal transition. These are differences worth noting as you advocate for yourself with doctors. Many physicians are unaware of how race and ethnicity can play into a patient's encounter with perimenopausal symptoms. Whether your symptoms fit into the expected timeline or not, they need to be taken seriously.

Given all these factors—environment, aging, life, your own unique body—perimenopause can look and feel different to each person, and it's important to keep all of them in mind as you read on. But there are certain similarities to what's happening in all our bodies. Let's get to our anatomy lesson.

2

The Hormonal Life Cycle

From First Period to Last and Everything In Between

Aren't hormones what make you mad?

—EIGHT-YEAR-OLD DAUGHTER OF A PERIMENOPAUSAL WOMAN

The sound of slamming doors was never a prominent acoustic feature in the home where Liane, forty-five, lived with her thirteen-year-old daughter, Maddie. Then, suddenly, it was, along with a lot of yelling. Liane, for her part, had recently been feeling grumpy, overly emotional, and very quick to anger. One look at the mess in Maddie's room would send her into a spiral of rage. Maddie, too, was grumpy, overly emotional, and quick to anger. While Liane was perplexed by how to navigate life on eggshells with a new teenager, the deeper cause of their clashes wasn't difficult to pinpoint: They were both suffering from hormonal chaos. And when perimenopause and puberty coincide in the same household—as they often do—it's double the trouble.

As Liane and Maddie can attest, any changes in the balance of hormones in the body can wreak havoc—whether they are rooted in puberty or perimenopause (the two can be so similar that perimenopause is sometimes referred to as a "second puberty"). So, when you find yourself in the throes of tumultuous and sometimes torturous symptoms, it can help to understand what hormones are, what they do, and how they change over one's lifespan.

Hormones don't rule everything in our lives, but they certainly play a starring role. That's because they do more than just regulate your menstrual cycle; they are chemical messengers that communicate important information across every bodily system. For instance, the thyroid hormones, secreted by the thyroid gland, tell the cells how quickly or slowly to use energy (this is what's known as your metabolism). Sex hormones, also known as reproductive hormones, are largely responsible for regulating sexual characteristics and the reproductive system. An example of that is follicle-stimulating hormone (FSH), a hormone made in the brain. In women, FSH tells the ovaries to begin growing an egg for potential fertilization; in men, it stimulates sperm production in the testes. But sex hormones don't just communicate with the reproductive organs; they influence everything from mental health to bone strength to how luxurious (or thinning) your hair is. Sex hormones, in other words, are the main physiological culprits behind perimenopausal symptoms and the ones we'll talk about most in this book.

The Perimenopause Players: Estrogen, Progesterone, and Testosterone

Estrogen

This hormone is made primarily in the ovaries, with small amounts produced in the adrenal glands (which sit on top of the kidneys) and by body fat. There are estrogen receptors all over your body—little structures inside and outside cells where estrogen can "dock" and pass on signals. Each estrogen receptor is only receptive to a particular type or types of estrogen, and depending on where the receptors live in the cell (inside, outside, in the nucleus), the estrogen has a different effect.

Estrogen's main role in reproduction is to help prompt ovulation—the release of an egg from the ovary for potential fertilization—and to help make a fluffy lining in the uterine wall where a fertilized egg can attach and grow. But estrogen also influences everything from blood flow, cholesterol levels, and the production of structural cells like collagen and elastin, to the pH environment in the body, the activity of bone cells, and the suppression of free radicals (rogue oxygen molecules that can damage DNA). It's through these and many other actions that estrogen affects the health of your heart, bones, skin and hair, pelvic muscles, and brain. As you'll see when we begin talking about individual symptoms and health risks later in the book, there is almost always an estrogen (or lack of estrogen) component at work.

There are four types of estrogen: estrone (E1), estradiol (E2), estriol (E3), and estetrol (E4). Estradiol (E2) is the type of estrogen made by the cells in your ovaries and a few other tissues. It's the one with the greatest responsibility in the body and is the most "potent" of the four. Estriol (E3) is made by the placenta to support a growing fetus; your body only makes it when you're pregnant. Estrone (E1) is made by the fat cells, and it becomes more dominant once you're in menopause and the ovaries cease making estradiol. (Estrone and other types of estrogen can be converted by the body tissues to estradiol.) Estetrol (E4) is made by the fetal liver during pregnancy, and it's used in some birth control pills.

It's not important that you memorize any of this information, but having some familiarity with the various types of estrogen may help you understand different hormone therapy options a little better. Estradiol is the predominant hormone used in menopausal hormone therapy (formerly known as hormone replacement therapy, or HRT, but we'll use "menopausal hormone therapy" and "MHT" in this book). We will discuss hormone therapy in more detail in part 3.

Progesterone

Like estrogen, progesterone is primarily produced in the ovaries. Its role in the reproductive system is to stabilize the lining of the uterus, as well as to tell it when to stop growing. Estrogen tells the uterine lining to grow; progesterone tells these new uterus-padding cells to stay put and also halts the growth operation. (If these cells were to continuously accumulate, it would increase the risk of developing precancer, and later, cancer.) When an egg is released but is not fertilized, progesterone levels drop, causing the lining of the uterus to break down and the body to shed it. This is your period.

Apart from its reproductive duties, progesterone has a soothing effect on the brain. In fact, it increases the production of the feel-good chemicals dopamine and gamma-aminobutyric acid (GABA). This is why some (but not all) women have a mood response—depression, anxiety, irritability, anger—to the perimenopausal rise and fall of progesterone. We don't know why, but some people are simply more sensitive to progesterone fluctuations than others.

Perimenopause is characterized by major highs and lows in progesterone, but eventually progesterone levels will fall to zero. By the time you reach full menopause, the body no longer produces progesterone. This makes sense, because progesterone's role in the reproductive cycle is to prepare you to implant an egg. So, if you're not making an egg, it's an out-of-work hormone, and the cells that make it have all died off, too. (Incidentally, this is why some people are encouraged to take progesterone during early pregnancy in the hopes that it will help the fertilized egg implant in the uterine wall, and lower the risk of miscarriage.) Sometimes one of us will get a request from a patient who, prompted by another healthcare provider, wants us to check their progesterone levels. But if you're in menopause, there's no reason to spend money on a progesterone test; it will almost always register at zero.

Progestogens (compounds that include progesterone and other similar molecules called progestins) are components of hormonal birth control and can be used alongside estradiol as part of a regimen of MHT. We'll talk more about the therapeutic use of progestogens as well as the differences between hormonal birth control and MHT in part 3.

Testosterone

Like estrogen, testosterone is made in many places in the body, including in the ovaries, in the adrenal glands, in the skin and muscle cells, and in the brain. Testosterone is a precursor to estrogen, meaning that it can be transformed into estrogen by an enzyme called aromatase. But other than that, it does not have a role in the egg-producing part of the reproductive cycle. It doesn't affect your period or ovulation or play a part in pregnancy.

Over the course of your lifetime, your testosterone level will gradually fall. Testosterone peaks in the twenties, then slowly declines, falling most precipitously when you're in your eighties. Contrary to what's often thought (and promoted by purveyors of testosterone therapies—see page 109), it does not go off a cliff during perimenopause or menopause. While the ovaries cease their function in relation to the menstrual cycle, ovulation, and estrogen production by the time you reach menopause, they continue to produce testosterone. In fact, some women in perimenopause experience increasingly available levels of testosterone. This isn't because you're making more testosterone, but because without estrogen, testosterone becomes more bioavailable in the body.

Typically, testosterone is held captive by a big molecule called sex hormone binding globulin (SHBG), which circulates in your blood and transports several hormones, holding them inactive until needed. SHBG soaks up testosterone like a sponge and keeps some of it from being used alongside estrogen. But when estrogen declines, so does SHBG. Fewer "sponges" means more testosterone left free to roam and be read by your cells. This is why many people experience things like acne, chin hairs, loss of hair on your head, and weight gain in your middle—typically things associated with men or testosterone—during perimenopause and beyond.

Another common misconception is that testosterone is central to a woman's libido. It actually has very little to do with sexual desire for most women. Testosterone is important for maintaining muscle mass and bone strength, and it helps keep vaginal and vulvar tissues healthy, both of which are important to consider during this time. But libido? Not so influential. We'll talk more about testosterone and sex drive in chapter 7.

Your Reproductive System in Three Acts

The sequence of events leading up to, during, and after perimenopause is all in service to building up, maintaining, then winding down your body's reproductive machinery (as perhaps goes without saying, whether you actually ever make a baby or not). You probably already know the basics of how your reproductive system works, but we're going to do a deeper dive here with the goal of helping you understand the underlying causes of all those crazy perimenopausal symptoms—from those three-pads-an-hour periods to the sleepless nights and newly formed belly fat. Being well-versed in the mechanics of the reproductive system can also give you considerable insight into the mechanics of your human self above and beyond perimenopause. So, let's take it from the top, before you were even born.

From Zero to Puberty

As you might imagine, a human egg is minuscule. It's about the size of a grain of salt, the tiny classic type of salt that sprinkles out of a saltshaker. The process by which female fetuses develop eggs (oocytes) begins as early as week seven of gestation, when the cells that will become eggs migrate into the developing ovaries. By month five, as many as 7 million eggs have been created through a special type of cell division. Usually when cells divide, they fully split in two and each new cell gets a complete copy of all the original cell's genetic material. Oocytes are different. They only partially divide during gestation and when they do divide all the way (which happens later, during ovulation), they only get half the chromosomes—the other half will be provided by the sperm cells during fertilization. This is important to remember because this unique type of cell division will come back to haunt us during perimenopause.

So, imagine yourself as a baby in utero, a maturing fetus with 7 million eggs. What happens to all of them? Most of those eggs won't meet the high standard nature sets for a fertilizable oocyte; only the "strong" will survive. The rest will die off and you'll end up with 1 to 2 million eggs when you're born—the highest number you'll ever have because you won't make any more eggs, and you'll even lose more of them over time. Through that same Darwinian, survival-of-the-fittest system that governed the eggs in utero, during a lifetime, the body will reject and reabsorb more than half of that 1 to 2 million pool of oocytes. But you don't need all those eggs; you just need enough of the good ones. On average, a woman will release (ovulate) only 400 to 500 eggs during her fertile years.

In childhood, the eggs remain stored in your ovaries in a state of partial development, each one tucked inside a bundle of cells called a follicle. And that's where they stay until you hit puberty and hormonal changes spur physical developments and set in motion the process that will allow you to conceive. Most girls go through puberty and get their first period anywhere from age nine to age thirteen. This is when the brain begins signaling the ovaries to start readying some of those partially developed eggs for possible fertilization. While we can identify the brain chemicals that signal the ovaries to snap into action, nobody has really figured out why the brain says, "It's go time!" when it does.

When all systems are go, the menstrual cycle and ovulation process begins. In the first part of the cycle, the hypothalamus gland in your brain releases a messenger called gonadotropin-releasing hormone (GnRH). GnRH is a versatile messenger that pulses through the body at different intervals and times of day in order to send distinct messages. To light up the monthly menstrual cycle, GnRH pulses in a pattern that tells the brain to release yet another messenger, this one the aforementioned FSH. FSH's job is to instruct the ovaries to take some of the eggs they've been warehousing and start growing them into maturity. These dormant eggs, as you might remember, are each encased in a follicle, and it's the follicles that support the progressive development of the eggs into potential candidates for fertilization.

Follicles also have other functions, among them, producing estrogen. As the designated clutch of eggs—about a dozen of them—mature, the follicles begin secreting estrogen. After a few days, one egg will emerge as the star candidate, becoming bigger and better than the rest. That superior egg's follicle will produce even more estrogen, which sends a message back to the brain: "We have a winner; no need to keep urging the ovaries to develop more eggs." This added secretion of estrogen from the viable egg's follicle also helps turn the normally thin walls of the uterine cavity into a nice, fluffy place to implant a fertilized egg and host a baby. It's this "fluffy" lining, made of blood and tissue, that, when shed, becomes your period.

At this time, another message gets sent to the brain, prompting it to send a substance known as luteinizing hormone (LH) down the ovaries' way. LH begins the next phase of your cycle by triggering the release of the "star" egg from its follicle. (On occasion, two eggs will emerge as victors, both will get released, and increase the chance of fraternal twins.) The egg will then move into the abdomen so a fallopian tube can collect it and where it can be available should any sperm cells wander by. The two, now joined in an elementary form of an embryo, then travel to the uterus and settle into its lining.

Luteinizing hormone also prompts the production of yet another hormone, progesterone. While the egg has left the follicle, the follicle still has a role to play here and that's the production of progesterone. Earlier in the cycle, estrogen built up the uterine lining; now progesterone comes along to stabilize it, feathering the bed with something akin to 700 thread-count sheets. But the body will only produce progesterone for a limited time. If fertilization occurs, the early placenta will take over progesterone production, ensuring that the uterus remains a hospitable place for the fetus. But if no fertilization occurs, the egg dies off, the follicle recedes, and progesterone levels abate. It's that drop in progesterone that tells your body it's time to shed the unused uterine lining and, fourteen days after the egg first dropped, your period will begin.

That last part of the cycle is pretty much fixed at fourteen days. The earlier phase, the part where you're building up the eggs in order to send that one best-in-class oocyte down the chute, can be somewhat variable, which accounts for why some women have longer cycles than others. The average menstrual cycle, though, is twenty-eight days.

Puberty to Perimenopause

After the irregularities of puberty quiet down, the reproductive system generally begins to work quite elegantly, like a well-played game of telephone with a series of hormones passing along messages in an orderly fashion to create a new human life. And, absent any reproductive disorders or anomalies, it can operate smoothly for years. But just like every other part of your body, your reproductive system is aging—and the remaining eggs in your ovaries are showing it. Now when your brain sends FSH down to prompt the preparation of eggs for ovulation, there's not a lot to work with. These eggs have been lying dormant for years and like a lot of that stuff you've had stored in your garage for decades, they begin to deteriorate.

Remember how earlier we said that when oocytes are first formed during gestation, they only divide their genetic material partway, waiting to split the rest of their genetic material during ovulation? After twenty or so years of suspended animation, it becomes more difficult for the eggs to faithfully divide the chromosomes, leading to a lot of dysfunctional eggs, most not worthy of ovulation. Those that are subpar but do make it through and are ultimately fertilized increase the risk of miscarriage or genetic anomalies. That's why it's harder to maintain a pregnancy when you're past your prime fertility years (in most women fertility begins a sharp decline in the early thirties), and the risks increase through your forties.

So, in perimenopause, here you are with eggs not quite up to snuff and, while the ovaries will respond to FSH's prompting to prepare a batch for ovulation, it doesn't always go well; it's a roller-coaster situation. Some months everything will proceed seamlessly, and the ovary will signal back to the brain, "Look, I found this good egg; all is well." And just a reminder: That good egg can be fertilized. You can still get pregnant during perimenopause!

But other months, the ovaries get the FSH signal only to find that the eggs they've recruited in response are mediocre. What often happens then is that, while the follicles do the work of bringing eggs to maturity, none of the oocytes will ever become suitable for ovulation. The brain, though, doesn't give up, intensifying the supply of FSH to keep signaling the ovaries to develop another batch of eggs.

Just a short detour here to give you a picture of what this looks like. The ovaries are little orbs, yet the eggs are actually not inside as you'd expect, but on the surface. If an ovary is like the earth, the eggs nestled in their follicles are the crust. Inside the ovaries is where other cells like testosterone are made. When the eggs are developing, they develop in place on top of the orb; then the "good" one gets released from the ovary.

So, during perimenopause, the brain is signaling the ovaries to keep going. Now you've got an accumulation of eggs in development, which, imperfect as they are, still release estrogen from the follicles supporting them, sending your estrogen levels soaring. After 30, 60, maybe even 90 days, all this work going on in your ovaries bears fruit: One of the eggs triumphs and you ovulate. Fourteen days later, if there is no fertilization, you will get your much-delayed period. And because you've been releasing so much estrogen, and estrogen builds up the lining of the uterus, once that big fat lining is shed and bleeding begins, it will be very, very heavy. There may be occasions when you actually don't ovulate, but you have a period anyway (the lining buildup becomes unstable and just starts to shed) with the same results: a veritable flood of blood.

Irregular or heavy bleeding is a signature of perimenopause. What was once a nicely synchronized system is now chaos. You will have those estrogen highs, but you will also have estrogen lows. During those times when your body is struggling to produce an egg worthy of ovulation, it is also making no progesterone. Remember, it's progesterone's role to prepare the uterus for implantation of an embryo, but if you go months without ovulating, there's no need for it. That means the soothing effect that progesterone has on the brain (at least in some women) will be absent, so that may be why you feel moody or even struggle with depression and anxiety at this time. The brain relishes a regular pattern; it does not like instability, so, all in all, these massive fluctuations of hormones are going to make you feel crummy and contribute to the symptoms we'll detail in chapters 4 through 12.

Perimenopause to Menopause

When you're in perimenopause and FSH comes knocking, your ovaries respond. As we just recounted, sometimes it takes them a while to eke out an acceptable egg, but they can do it. In menopause, when the brain sends FSH to the ovaries, it gets no response. Then, like a toddler who can't get his mother's attention, the brain yells louder by prompting the production of more FSH. But the brain's "C'mon, ovaries, there's got to be one more!" is met with radio silence. Since nothing is happening, no estrogen is being secreted from follicles around developing eggs. Because estrogen is also made in small amounts in the fat cells and adrenal glands, you won't be running on empty, but you've now reached two of the hormonal hallmarks of menopause: high FSH and low estrogen levels.

That may sound ominous, but as the hormonal fits and starts and the all-around unpredictability of perimenopause come to an end, menopause is when things actually calm down. Sure, it has its own travails, including some health challenges that we'll cover in part 4. But it's hopefully a consolation to know that you can look forward to the return of some sense of normality. Right now, though, nothing may seem normal. In the next chapters, we'll address what to do about it.

Part Two

All Changes, Great and Small

3

Erratic Periods

Coping with the Ebbs and Flows

Otherwise, it looks like a murder scene in my house . . .

—PERIMENOPAUSAL PATIENT ON TAKING EXTREME
STEPS TO STEM MENSTRUAL BLEEDING

The dress was chosen with care, a long sheath made of cream-colored antique lace worn over a satin slip. Elegant and timeless, perfectly suited to the bride, Elena. After posing for photographs with family, she and her sister retreated to the dressing room. Climbing the back stairs of the old building where Elena and her husband-to-be would soon be married before a crowd of 150 people, her alarmed sister asked, "What's that on the back of your dress?"

You can see where this is heading. It was blood, menstrual overflow. At forty-two, Elena had had her period many times before. It was annoying (*of course* she had to have her period on her wedding day), but today wasn't the first day, and it had never been particularly heavy. With guests and her fiancé waiting, she quickly rinsed the blood out, used the usual tampon, and didn't give it another thought. "When I think back, I wonder what I would have done if, for some reason, I had not calmly gone into a zen state, took off the dress, doused it with water in the sink, and blown it dry with a hair dryer," remembers Elena. "I had it back on in perfect condition within fifteen minutes." While it thankfully didn't interrupt her wedding, this unexpected overflow was one of the first signs for Elena of perimenopause and the attendant changes to her body.

Unpredictable periods are a classic symptom of perimenopause, and often one of the first telltale signs that this process has begun. Once upon a time, you may have only had to worry about whether wearing white pants after Labor Day is a fashion faux pas, not whether they're going to get stained red. Now that you're in perimenopause, you may find yourself doing things you haven't done since you were a high school freshman, like always bringing along a sweater to wrap around your waist, just in case you bleed through. You've entered a time of menstrual unpredictability. Your period can be unexpectedly heavier. It can be lighter. It can be shorter. It can be longer. Your cycles can be spaced out. They can be closer together. They can be more painful. They can be less painful (bonus!). Any or all of those changes are possible, without any apparent rhyme or reason.

What It Feels Like and Why

While most women are aware that one day in the future they'll stop menstruating and therefore be in menopause, many of us are unprepared for the inconsistencies and sometimes scary changes that can lead up to the period shutoff. While 14 to 25 percent of premenopausal women have cycles that are either shorter or longer than the average, the majority of women spend years having you-can-set-your-watch-by-it periods, so the sudden fluctuations brought on by perimenopause can be unsettling. Is something wrong? Take our word for it, in most cases, this is all par for the course.

Variability is a hallmark of perimenopausal periods, but the progress of these changes often follows a common pattern. The first thing that typically occurs is a change in cycle length, with periods getting closer together. Cycle length refers to the first day of one period to the first day of the next period. In most women, the menstrual cycle is a 28-day series of reproductive events: egg recruitment and development, building up of the uterus lining, egg release (ovulation), then 14 days later (if no fertilization takes place), the uterus sheds its lining and bleeding begins. In perimenopause, that 28-day cycle may shorten to 23 or 24 days. You'll think, *Didn't I just have my period?* And then, lo and behold, there it is again. And having these closely spaced periods can go on for years, which is typical if somewhat bothersome. Throughout perimenopause, the process of hormone signaling—how the brain talks to your ovaries—is in flux, and these menstrual shifts are symptoms of the hormonal changes the body is experiencing.

What usually transpires next—typically when you're within a year or two of your last period—is that the cycle changes from being shorter, with periods closer together, to longer, so they become more spaced out. As you get nearer to menopause, you may even go three or four months without periods. And when you do get them, they may be very heavy. As you might remember from chapter 2, during the three to four months between periods, your ovaries are still trying (and trying) to grow an egg viable enough to be released for ovulation. Over that span of time you might not get a period, but estrogen is still being released by the final, striving eggs, which causes the lining of the uterus to thicken far more than it would during a normal cycle. It's like when you go on vacation and forget to cancel your newspaper delivery. The delivery driver doesn't know to stop, so the papers pile up until you come home and throw them in the recycling. Without either an embryo or a message telling it to shed, the uterine lining keeps building up, just like those papers.

When the message finally comes and you do get your period, all that extra lining causes the kind of flood that can unexpectedly soil a wedding dress—or worse. Some women find that perimenopausal periods can be so heavy that they start to disrupt normal life. Natalie was a patient of Amy's who would stay home the first two days of her period wearing an adult diaper because she bled so hard. But even that wasn't enough to prevent leaking, so she'd get into the bathtub with her laptop and do her work in the tub. Women—we solve problems! (But that isn't the way to solve that particular problem, which we'll get to later in this chapter.)

This is the typical pattern—a cycle that gets shorter and then longer throughout perimenopause—but of course not everyone's body follows a "typical" trajectory. We've had patients who had 100 percent regular periods throughout perimenopause. Every 28 days, exactly the same consistency, exactly the same pain level, and then their periods stopped, and they never had one again. We have had patients who bleed only every four to six months for five years, and each time there's that big gap, they think, *This is the last one*, only to bleed again (often at the most inconvenient times). You should talk to your doctor as you go through these changes, but know that menstruation in perimenopause can look different for everyone.

Another symptom some people experience during perimenopause is bleeding and/or pain during ovulation. This has a lovely German name, "mittelschmerz," which means "middle pain" because it typically occurs on the fourteenth day—the middle—of the menstrual cycle. The pain is thought to be caused by fluid, secreted by the follicle when an egg is released for ovulation, and irritating to the abdomen. Some women experience pain while ovulating before perimenopause, but it's not uncommon to begin experiencing it for the first time during this volatile time. Mittelschmerz is considered "referred pain," which means that the brain has received a signal that there's a problem, but it's creating pain somewhere other than the trouble spot. In this case, the pain is felt on one side of the abdomen, which can make it feel like you're having appendicitis. This is something Rebecca knows firsthand, having panicked that she was having an "appendicitis" every 60 days or so until she realized it was mittelschmerz. (Yes, we physicians sometimes freak out, too.)

What You Can Do About It

We always recommend talking to your doctor before trying to remedy erratic and/or heavy periods on your own. Even though some amount of menstrual volatility is to be expected during the perimenopausal years, we always want to do a workup on our patients just to make sure there isn't anything else going on. The hormonal volatility of perimenopause can make relatively benign conditions, like fibroids, worse. We also want to make sure that the erratic periods themselves aren't causing any problems. The main period-related conditions we want to keep an eye on during this time are fibroids, adenomyosis, and polyps or other potentially precancerous lesions in the uterus, though of course your doctor may flag other things to keep an eye on based on your personal history.

During their childbearing years, 70 to 80 percent of all women will develop fibroids—benign balls of muscle cells and connective tissue in the wall of the uterus. If you're Black, this is extra important to be aware of, because research shows that Black women develop fibroids at a higher rate than white women, and they're often larger, too. Most of the time, fibroids are totally harmless, and you might not even notice they're there. But during perimenopause, irregular hormone signaling from the brain can cause them to grow erratically, impacting the uterus's ability to regulate blood flow and causing heavy bleeding.

Normally, the uterus slows bleeding by contracting and clamping down on the blood vessels. That's the cause of menstrual cramps—the clamping down denies oxygen to the uterus, which generates cramping and pain. But when fibroids get in the way, the floodgates open, and this can lead to excessive bleeding. Fibroids can also get into the cavity of the uterus and that, too, can cause a heavy menstrual flow.

Another problem we look for with heavy menstrual bleeding is adenomyosis, a condition in which small pouches develop in the uterus where the built-up uterine lining gets caught. When it comes time to shed the lining, the uterus has trouble pushing it out of these little cul-de-sacs, and it causes a lot of cramping and pain. When the lining does finally get out, it can cause the kind of three-maxi-pad alarm that makes you consider buying stock in Kotex. There's also a risk that losing so much blood at once can cause anemia.

Uterine polyps and precancerous lesions can occur in anyone with a uterus, but they are much more likely to occur in perimenopause and menopause than at any other time. When hormone levels are seesawing, the uterine lining thickens unchecked, which can lead to precancerous cells. Polyps can also develop in the uterus during this time, and as you get older, there's an increased risk that they can be cancerous. Most often, polyps and other growths are benign, but these different kinds of growths can cause intermenstrual bleeding—or bleeding between periods—as well as pain or bleeding during sex. Polyps, fibroids, precancerous lesions—any of these types of structural issues—can get irritated if they're "bumped" into during intercourse. So, that's something your doctor should want to evaluate, too.

If you were one of our patients, we'd want you to come in if you're experiencing any of these scenarios: skipping periods, then having really heavy ones; bleeding more frequently; bleeding uncontrollably for several days; or having a lot of bleeding in between periods. Intermenstrual bleeding can occur when you're ovulating irregularly because the lining, built up from so many tries at growing a viable egg, is unstable.

But it can also be a sign of other issues, such as polyps in the endometrium or the cervix as well other places in the reproductive system. It's always worth talking to your doctor if there is a bleeding change. This goes for bleeding after sex as well, if that's something new. Most of the time irregular bleeding is just irregular bleeding, part of the perimenopausal roller coaster. But don't be alarmed if your doctor wants to do some tests just to be confident that it's only perimenopause causing your symptoms.

During the Checkup

When a perimenopausal patient comes in with any kind of erratic bleeding, we generally start a workup with an ultrasound. An ultrasound, as you might know, is a painless imaging procedure that gives a snapshot of your uterus. In this context (as, say, opposed to during pregnancy) we use it to see how thick the lining of the uterus is, and whether there are fibroids or polyps present. A thicker lining may indicate an overgrowth of tissue, a hidden polyp, or, less likely, precancerous or cancerous cells. The next step, if necessary, would be to retrieve a sample of uterine tissue through a biopsy. (Another thing to note if you're a Black woman: Studies show that Black women have a higher incidence of cancer in the lining of the uterus even at normal thickness, so we usually recommend that our Black patients have a biopsy, even if the ultrasound is normal.)

When we do a biopsy, we're generally looking for precancer and cancer cells as well as signs of fibroids or polyps. Biopsies involve inserting an instrument through the vagina and cervix and into the uterus to retrieve a tissue sample. They're typically quick office procedures, and while they can make you crampy, they don't generally require anesthesia. That said, don't be afraid to ask your doctor for pain management if you think it could be of benefit to you. Some women find uterine biopsies very uncomfortable, and there are several ways to lessen the discomfort, including using a numbing medication like lidocaine gel in the vagina or a lidocaine injection in the cervix (it's called a paracervical block). Other options include oral narcotics, anti-inflammatories, and/or anti-anxiety medications. Some offices are even able to offer nitrous oxide "laughing gas" or intravenous medication similar to a colonoscopy. There is the option of having the procedure in an operating room (OR) with anesthesia, too.

If preliminary tests like the ultrasound and biopsy show the presence of a very thick lining, polyps, or fibroids, we'll also likely recommend a hysteroscopy for further evaluation. Despite the fact that it sounds like "hysterectomy," hysteroscopy is a much simpler procedure. It involves going through the vagina and cervix into the uterus with a tiny camera attached to a thin tube. (Amy describes it to her patients as being like a "colonoscopy without a bowel prep.") If we find something while we're in there, we can also use a tool to remove any abnormalities, which can help put an end to excessive bleeding—it's akin to a little Pac Man that sucks the abnormal tissue out. In most cases, the whole thing gets wrapped up within a few minutes. And unlike the biopsy, a hysteroscopy is always done with anesthesia, either in the office or in the OR.

Treatment Options

A patient comes in and says, "My period is so heavy now. I bleed for five days and have to wear a maxi pad on the heaviest day." "A maxi pad every hour?" "No, a maxi pad the whole day." It doesn't sound that bad, does it? To some women, one maxi pad a day might be nothing. But to the patient who had this conversation with Rebecca, it was a totally new experience, unexpectedly arising after years of fairly light bleeding. Change, no matter where it falls on a scale of 1 to 10, can be distressing. If it feels weird, it is weird, and there's no shame in wanting to understand such a drastic change. Sometimes you might want to see your doctor just to get some reassurance that, yes, what's happening is in line with what's expected at your age. Then you can decide if you want to do something about your period or not.

And if you do, there are several things you can try. The simplest is ibuprofen. Taking a big dose, 600 to 800 mg every eight hours, can help lighten the bleeding somewhat. And it will certainly help with cramps. This is your best over-the-counter bet. Doing this for one to three days during a period is fine, but if you're doing this every day, it can impact your kidneys. Talk to your doctor if you are taking ibuprofen frequently. Another option is a prescription drug called tranexamic acid (brand name Lysteda). It's FDA (Food and Drug Administration)-approved for uterine bleeding and works by slowing the breakdown of blood clots. You only need to take it for one to five days, during the heaviest part of menstruation. It won't change the frequency of your periods, but it will decrease the blood flow. Big asterisk: If you have a history of blood clots or are taking oral hormones containing estrogen, you're not a candidate for tranexamic acid.

Birth control pills are a great option for managing erratic and heavy bleeding. The most proactive way to find relief from erratic periods is to make them stop altogether with a continuous regimen of birth control pills; but even taking pills cyclically can help reduce bothersome bleeding. There are many variations on birth control pills, giving you a lot of options. They're safe for most women, and they can help treat a range of other symptoms of perimenopause. Another way to lighten bleeding is to get a hormonal intrauterine device (IUD). We'll provide more details on the use of birth control for perimenopause in chapter 13.

There are a few more pharmaceutical solutions worth mentioning. One is leuprolide (brand name Lupron), a shot, that's often used to shrink fibroids and other tissue, which can help with bleeding and pelvic pain. Elagolix and Relugolix are both tablets that have a similar effect but work in a different way: They block the pulsing pattern of gonadotropin-releasing hormone (GnRH) in the brain (see page 34). The downside of these medications is that they put you into temporary menopause. That may not be a problem if you're already close, but if you've got a ways to go, it may trigger an abrupt onset of menopausal symptoms that you're not quite ready for.

The remedies we recommend to patients depend on what we're trying to fix. If it's just bleeding, we might offer one suggestion. If it's bleeding and mood symptoms, we might propose another. There are a lot of factors that we take into account when counseling perimenopausal patients. And sometimes there's some trial and error involved. Amy started Natalie, the patient who had taken to her bathtub to control bleeding, on a birth control pill to see if it would help (and it was easy to start right away). But because her periods were unusually heavy, Amy made sure to keep a few other options in her back pocket just in case. Luckily, the pill worked fabulously, and Natalie's bathtub went back to being a place for bathing.

Although Natalie's case was successful on the first try, we don't want to mislead you about how easy it might be to figure out what works. Different people respond differently to various treatments, so it's not unusual to have to try a few to get optimal results. Sometimes birth control pills don't stop the bleeding, and we'll have to combine them with an IUD or IUD and tranexamic acid. There's an art to the science of treating perimenopause, so don't give up if the first go-round isn't a triumph. Talking to your doctor can help you hone in on a treatment that works best for you.

Other Kinds of Interventions

When bleeding is beyond the control of a prescription, if someone is for whatever reason not a candidate for hormone treatments, or we know that there's a structural issue exacerbating bleeding, there are surgical options. The hysteroscopy we mentioned earlier can take care of some types of polyps or some of the fibroids that heighten bleeding. After that procedure, you may not need to do anything more. There's also something called an endometrial or uterine ablation, which involves removing a layer of the lining of the uterus through various methods (among them heat, cold, radio frequency or microwaves, and electricity). This procedure does have a few downsides. It causes scarring in the uterine cavity, so if it fails, you can't use an IUD to help with bleeding, and it makes it more difficult to check for cancerous tissue in the future. It's also only done on women who don't plan on becoming pregnant. You can technically still become pregnant after an ablation, but it will be a dangerous pregnancy because the scarring can lead to an abnormal attachment of your placenta, causing a life-threatening condition. So we consider it more of a last resort than the options previously discussed.

Another surgical procedure your doctor may mention is a uterine artery embolization (also called a uterine fibroid embolization). This is done by an interventional radiologist and involves placing substances in the arteries leading to the fibroids, thereby blocking the blood supply and effectively shrinking the offending structures. The procedure can decrease the bleeding enough so that it's tolerable, but because it can interrupt blood flow to the ovaries as well as the uterus and fibroids, uterine artery embolization can lead to a decrease in ovarian function and therefore hasten menopause (by a few months). So it's another option, but it doesn't have as high of a success rate as some of the other procedures we mentioned, and women with large fibroids may experience significant pain afterward.

Other options involve removing the cause of excess blood flow entirely, whether that means taking out the fibroids or the whole uterus. A myomectomy is a surgical procedure that removes large fibroids that may be growing in the wall of the uterus while still preserving the uterus, so it's an option for women who still want to get pregnant. For women who no longer want the potential of pregnancy, a hysterectomy is an option, especially for those who are really struggling with bleeding and haven't found a way to make it stop. A hysterectomy involves the complete removal of the uterus, but the gynecologic surgeon can leave the ovaries behind so you still make estrogen and the menopausal transition will proceed naturally. There are now many minimally invasive ways to perform a hysterectomy, and most women recover quickly from the surgery.

ENDOMETRIOSIS AND PERIMENOPAUSE

Some of the symptoms of perimenopause—heavy or irregular periods, pelvic pain, fatigue—are also symptoms of endometriosis. Two to 10 percent of women between the ages of twenty-five and forty are affected by endometriosis, which occurs when endometrial cells that make up the lining (interior) of the uterus grow outside the uterus, elsewhere in the body. As the endometrial cells spread throughout the reproductive and abdominal area (they can also sometimes grow in places like the lungs and brain), they can develop into big cysts, scar tissue, or adhesions that cause the organs to stick together. This often results in pelvic pain, pain during sex, the aforementioned bad periods, and fatigue, as well as infertility. And perimenopause can make everything worse because it's a time when you're getting a lot more hormone stimulation, encouraging the proliferation of endometrial cells.

It's not easy to see endometriosis on an ultrasound; it might be noticeable on an MRI, but the best way to diagnose it is through laparoscopic surgery. And it can be a confounding condition because not everyone suffers through all the symptoms we mentioned above. Rebecca had a patient who had what would be considered stage 4 (the most severe type) endometriosis: Her uterus, fallopian tubes, and the bowel were all fused together with endometrial tissue. But this patient never had a day of pain. Rebecca found the endometriosis incidentally when trying to determine why the patient couldn't get pregnant. (After undergoing a complicated eight-hour surgery to address her endometriosis, she later successfully gave birth to a healthy baby.) On the other end of the spectrum are women who have horrible, debilitating pain each month despite only having a few very small lesions. We all experience pain differently and we all have different inflammatory responses to conditions in the body. And this goes for everything from how you might experience something like endometriosis to how you experience perimenopause.

The Importance of Iron

No matter what type of treatment you choose for heavy bleeding, and especially if you choose no treatment at all, make sure you're getting enough iron either through your diet or by taking an iron supplement. Heavy bleeding can lead to anemia, and anemia is a gateway to fatigue, hair loss, a racing heart, headaches, and muscle cramps. Iron-rich foods include red meat, pork, seafood, chicken, eggs, beans, dark leafy greens, sweet potatoes, broccoli, green beans, dried fruit, watermelon, strawberries, and iron-fortified breads and cereals. To maximize absorption, eat them in combination with foods high in vitamin C like citrus, tomatoes, and bell peppers. On the flip side, don't eat them with coffee, tea, or dairy products like milk or yogurt, all of which can interfere with absorption.

Iron supplements are also an effective antidote to anemia, but they can have some side effects. Some people find them nauseating since you need to swallow the pills on an empty stomach to ensure your body soaks up the iron. They can also cause constipation. Some research suggests that you can mitigate these side effects by taking iron supplements every other day instead of the usual suggested way (a half dose twice daily every day), and as a bonus, this may yield better absorption.

Experiencing heavier bleeding during perimenopause, as well as other irregularities in your cycle, is to be expected, but there are many ways to manage it. It's not abnormal to have to step up your purchase of feminine hygiene products, but it's not something you have to live with either. If the bleeding is impacting your quality of life, talk to your doctor about the different options available to make it stop or at least ease up. And, while most heavy menstrual bleeding and other changes during perimenopause are benign, it's always good to get an evaluation, just to be on the safe side.

4

Bad Night's Sleep

The Curse of the 2 A.M. Wake-Up Call

I had to start sleeping on my side because suddenly I had pain in my hips and knees. I kept waking up in the middle of the night anyway.

—FORTY-THREE-YEAR-OLD PERIMENOPAUSAL PATIENT

It had been a rough year. First, Katherine's father had died. Then, her serious long-distance relationship had ended. She was in the middle of a lawsuit against her employer, as her boss had created a hostile workplace. Now she was preparing to move away from Seattle, a city she loved, to be closer to her mom in Southern California. Inevitably, she was sleepless (yes, she really was "Sleepless in Seattle") and having a hard time holding it together. At forty-five, Katherine was also hitting perimenopause. Was it adding to her nighttime awakenings? It was hard to parse out. All she knew was that, despite having been a solid sleeper before this tornado of life events, she now needed Tylenol PM, and eventually Xanax to help her get enough rest to function the next day (and even these gave her a bit of a "hangover" effect, which wasn't so helpful).

Sleep is one of our most vulnerable and critically important systems; everyone regardless of age, gender, race, ethnicity, or personality needs quality sleep to stay healthy. And not only do we all need it; we all need lots of it. So much of the maintenance and repair work in our body occurs as we catch the proverbial forty winks that, if we don't spend enough time in the "shop," various systems start to break down. Insufficient sleep—for adults that's usually less than seven hours a night—inhibits the body's ability to correctly produce hormones, respond to insulin, mend the heart and blood vessels, and fight infection. As such, it can contribute to the development of heart disease, kidney disease, high blood pressure, diabetes, stroke, and obesity. If you spend hundreds of nights not sleeping well, it can take years off your life.

The brain, too, is very dependent on sleep for optimal functioning. While we're off in dreamland, the brain rejuvenates and consolidates learning and long-term memories. Sleep is also intimately associated with daily mental performance, which is probably unsurprising if you've ever pulled an all-nighter only to find you're a complete mess the next day. But even a little reduction in sleep over a long period of time can affect us. When we aren't regularly getting a solid seven hours (more or less—there's some variability among people), it becomes harder to make decisions, solve problems, and pay attention. We all know that toddlers have trouble holding it together when they don't get a nap, but the truth is that even adults are more likely to struggle to control their emotions and cope with change when they're sleep-deprived. Lack of sleep is also associated with mental health disorders like anxiety and depression.

If you created a Venn diagram with sleep deprivation issues in one circle and perimenopausal issues in another, there would be a great deal of overlap in the middle: brain fog, irritability, emotional lows, anxiety, and weight gain are just a few of the many symptoms connected to both. They can also exacerbate each other's symptoms. For instance, anxiety triggered by hormonal changes can contribute to sleep deficit, and sleep deficit can spark more anxiety. It's all one big muddle, which often makes it difficult to tease out what exactly is causing certain perimenopausal symptoms—is it lack of sleep, or hormonal changes, or both? Nonetheless, we do know for certain that sleep disturbances are far more common in midlife women than in men of the same age, so it's not just aging that's keeping women up at night: According to the National Institutes of Health, 39 to 47 percent of women report sleep disturbances in perimenopause, an increase from the 16 to 42 percent who have them premenopause. In this chapter we'll explore the potential causes of sleep difficulties during this stage, as well as some of the available solutions.

What It Feels Like and Why

"I have no trouble getting to sleep. I get in bed at nine, turn off the lights at ten, and am quickly fast asleep. Then at two or three in the morning I snap awake and my mind is racing. Thoughts are spinning around in my head and it's two hours before I can fall back asleep—if I fall back asleep at all. The next day I'm exhausted." We've heard this story from so many perimenopausal patients—it's a textbook scenario. Some women also have trouble falling asleep, but the middle-of-the-night wake-up is our patients' most common sleep complaint.

Normally, sleep comes in four stages of varying length, each characterized by different brain activity, and during a normal sleep window, you cycle through these stages as many as four to six times. The first three stages are different levels of non-rapid eye movement (NREM) sleep; the last stage is rapid eye movement (REM) sleep. During REM sleep, your muscles relax, your eyes move, your heart rate increases, and your brain is highly active. It's the stage of sleep when you dream the most vividly as well as consolidate memories and process things that you learned during the day. The first two stages of NREM sleep are relatively light, but the third stage is a deep sleep, characterized by slow waves in the brain. It's during this stage that your body repairs itself, shoring up its immune function and restoring muscle and bone in a natural cycle of cell turnover.

All these stages of sleep are integral to good health and mental agility, so interruptions to any of them can affect your well-being. But for women experiencing perimenopause, it's not always clear whether changes to sleep are related to the turbulence of this specific time or a consequence of aging in general. As noted in chapter 2, sleep patterns change as a matter of course with age, and both men's and women's amount of nighttime sleep declines each decade. As you grow older, elements that control the circadian rhythm—the twenty-four-hour cycle that governs the sleep-wake cycle, also known as the biological clock—decline, as does the production of cortisol and melatonin, two hormones instrumental in easing the way to a good night's sleep. That's why your grandfather is always drifting off in front of the TV at 8 p.m., padding around in the middle of the night, and waking before the birds, only to be napping a short time later. That's not generally a forty-year-old's problem, but during midlife, these sleep-related hormones are beginning to shift and may factor into sleep disturbances. Perimenopause on top of the age-related changes adds a whole separate set of circumstances to the mix.

There doesn't seem to be any consensus on what stage of sleep is most likely to be interrupted when a woman is in perimenopause, but there is some indication that anxiety—a symptom of perimenopause—can affect REM sleep by creating disturbing dreams that trigger waking. But anxiety, which we'll get to in a minute (and explore more fully in the next chapter), is not the only prime actor in insomnia, nor are night sweats: The SWAN study (see page 25) found that a convergence of factors both related and unrelated to perimenopause conspires to keep a preponderance of midlife women staring at the ceiling at night.

Let's start with the role sex hormones may play. When looking specifically at sleep, SWAN investigators found that perimenopausal women had more nighttime problems when estrogen swung wide from its baseline level, implying that bigger volatility in estrogen levels may cause sleep issues to occur or worsen. There may be a sleep–progesterone connection as well. Progesterone, also in flux during perimenopause, has hypnotic effects on the brain, or what researchers like to call an ability to decrease "neuronal excitability." That is, it's calming. Estrogen, like progesterone, can impact mood, though it has other effects that can contribute to sleep quality (or lack thereof) as well. Some animal research suggests that the midlife drop in estrogen may affect the body's circadian rhythm as well as how efficiently your body can adapt to sleep disruptors.

In one study, conducted by researchers at Bridgewater State University in Massachusetts and published in 2023, three groups of mice were exposed to constant light, known to unsettle the normal workings of the circadian rhythm. Two groups of mice had their ovaries surgically removed, and one of those two ovary-less groups was given an estrogen replacement. A third group of mice served as a control. At the study's end, only the mice with no source of estrogen had disorganized sleep. Instead of the normal eight-to-twelve-hour blocks of rest the mice were known for, the mice with no estrogen cycled in and out of periods of sleep and wakefulness. Obviously, we're not rodents (even if midlife can sometimes feel like being on a hamster wheel), but this study and others like it offer some clues to why perimenopausal women just can't stay asleep.

Racing Thoughts

Anxiety—whether it's due to midlife circumstances, hormonal fluctuations, or, most likely, a combination of both—contributes to wakefulness and the kind of racing thoughts that keep you awake once you're up. While we'll cover perimenopause-precipitated anxiety in detail in the next chapter, it bears mention in relation to sleep, and in particular to what might be called an anxiety–wakefulness vicious cycle: "Once a person experiences a poor night of sleep or a string of poor nights of sleep, they begin to feel fearful and have anticipatory anxiety about sleep," says Meredith Broderick, MD, a neurologist and sleep specialist in Seattle. When people change their behavior in response to anticipatory anxiety, they might accidentally disrupt sleep further and make insomnia worse. "They might, for instance, increase the time they spend in bed, which increases WASO—waking after sleep onset—and decreases sleep drive. They might also start to devote more time and attention to sleep, developing a willful attitude about it rather than letting it happen." Some things you can't force; you just need to let nature take its course.

Dr. Broderick points out another contributing factor in keeping perimenopausal women (and all women for that matter) awake at night: not anxiety exactly, but just a heavy mental load of external distractions drawing our attention. "We have almost no time for reflection, slow thinking, or to be alone with our thoughts. This time is a real requirement of the brain—we call it the default mode network. It's the reason creative people go to remote places to be alone so they can come up with big ideas. If our attention is occupied at every moment throughout the day, our brain performs this function—which can also include processing difficult emotions and stressors—when we're in bed." While there may be other factors affecting your ability to sleep well, managing anxiety often goes a long way in helping mitigate the effects of perimenopausal insomnia and the resulting sleep deficit.

Not Breathing Easy

Of course, anxiety isn't the only thing that can affect your rest during perimenopause. Obstructive sleep apnea can affect anyone, but your risk increases during perimenopause. In the United States, 25 percent of women are at risk for sleep apnea, and changing hormones often play a role. Sleep apnea is a disorder characterized by breathing that stops and starts many times as you slumber. The pauses might not even seem to rouse you, at least that you're conscious of (although it often causes snoring, which might wake up your bed partner). While you may not notice or remember these moments, the body does wake you up just enough to get you to breathe again. Waking up over and over again means that you're rarely able to reach the deep sleep stages you need to fully rest and refresh your body. If you feel extremely tired in the morning for no apparent reason, sleep apnea may be the culprit. As one patient, Beth, recounts, "I always slept well, but I was also always strangely exhausted. Then I went to see a cardiologist for a required checkup before I had a knee replacement and the doctor noticed that my blood pressure was way up. I did a home test using an app and a device and it turned out I had severe sleep apnea. I had no idea."

Because it decreases oxygen intake, sleep apnea can put you at greater risk of high blood pressure, diabetes, heart disease, and stroke. (It sets you up for so many complications that Dr. Broderick calls it "the emperor of all sleep disorders.") The likelihood of developing the disorder increases with age for both women and men, although men are three times as likely to experience it as women. Still, women's numbers edge up during the menopausal transition. According to the Sleep in Midlife Women Study, a research project at the University of Wisconsin, disordered breathing is 21 percent higher in perimenopausal women than in premenopausal women. And the incidence continues to climb during the menopausal transition, with each year related to a 4 percent rise in risk of sleep apnea. The researchers also found that the rise in risk was independent of aging, meaning that it's not just about getting older—it's due to risks specifically associated with perimenopause.

There are a few issues that come up during perimenopause that make sleep apnea risk rise. One is that you may be gaining weight, which substantially increases the likelihood of developing the condition. It may also have something to do with where you're gaining weight. During perimenopause and beyond, weight becomes more likely to accumulate in the upper body and therefore closer to the airway, a risk factor for sleep apnea. In that same vein, another potential risk factor is loss of muscle mass. One of the places we lose muscle mass is in our neck and throats, so we don't support the airway as well as we once may have. Declining progesterone can also complicate things. In some ways, this hormone is soporific. But in the respiratory system, progesterone is stimulating, so a drop in the hormone, some researchers have hypothesized, may have something to do with disordered breathing.

While body weight can be a risk factor, you don't have to be overweight to experience sleep apnea (nor are you guaranteed to experience sleep apnea if you are overweight). If you're chronically tired for no apparent reason, your doctor may suggest a sleep study, a diagnostic test that records several physiological processes while you sleep during the night. It's really the only way to diagnose the problem. Luckily, it doesn't have to be a big ordeal—you can actually do a sleep study at home, so you don't need to spend the night in a lab. Your doctor sends the machine out, you hook yourself up, and you get to do the test from your own bed. If you do find that you have sleep apnea, there are a variety of devices that can help, ranging from machines that provide pressure to the airways to keep it open (like the Continuous Positive Airway Pressure [CPAP] device) to dental devices.

The Heat Is On

One of the hallmarks of perimenopause is night sweats, which are caused by hot flashes during sleep (hot flashes around the clock are more common as you near menopause). Not everyone gets them, and they're certainly not the only cause of perimenopausal sleep disturbance. But, as those who do experience night sweats know, they can derail a good night's rest. The SWAN sleep and perimenopause study found that night sweats not only disrupt sleep but can also make it harder to fall back asleep and lead some women to wake early.

Temperature plays an important role in sleep. As part of the circadian rhythm, your body's core temperature begins dropping a couple of hours before you typically turn out the lights to prepare you to fall asleep. Sleepiness, helped along with the simultaneous release of the hormone melatonin, ensues. Your temperature remains lowered (about 2 degrees from your normal body temperature) through the night, then rises again toward waking. Night sweats and nighttime hot flashes throw a real wrench into this beautifully designed temperature calibration. Even if the rise in body temperature doesn't wake you up (although it probably will), it can lead to a decrease in restorative deep sleep. Heat has also been shown to decrease REM sleep. Any way you slice it, body temperature fluctuations at night impact how refreshed you feel the next day.

What You Can Do About It

We'll discuss some perimenopause-specific sleep tips later in this chapter, but the first step in managing sleep issues is something you've probably encountered before: basic sleep hygiene, the term for routines and behaviors that promote good sleep. These are relatively simple considerations, but they can make a big difference in how deeply and expansively you slumber through the night. Here are the main tenets:

> ➤ Be consistent in your timing. Try to go to bed at the same time each night and wake up at the same time each morning. The body loves a familiar pattern.

> ➤ Have a nighttime routine, like lowering the lights and reading for a while before turning in. Let your body ease into it.

> ➤ Turn off blue light–emitting devices like phones, computers, and tablets thirty to sixty minutes before bed. Blue light can inhibit sleep-inducing melatonin. Better yet, leave them in the other room

so that you aren't awakened by the pinging of texts from your best friend (who is also awake because she, too, is in perimenopause).

➤ Make your bed a sacred space, reserved for sleep and sex only. This will help make that Pavlovian connection: When you see your bed, it may even make you sleepy, or, well, you know (which may then lead to sleep).

➤ Cultivate daytime habits that promote good sleep, like exercise, exposure to daylight (get outside each day), and limiting caffeine to the earlier hours of the day.

➤ Create a good sleep environment by blocking noise and light (blackout shades are always good).

➤ Keep your room temperature, if possible, between a cool 65 and 68 degrees.

➤ Minimize drinking. Alcohol may seem like a great way to lull yourself to sleep, and it may even make you drowsy, but it makes it harder to get into deep sleep and can increase nighttime waking.

➤ If you simply can't sleep, it's better to get up for a bit than to force it. If you wake up and can't fall back asleep within twenty minutes, get out of bed and read in low light, stretch, meditate, or do something else that calms your mind (which probably isn't answering work emails and bathing in blue light at 3 a.m.).

But say you've followed all these rules and you're still struggling. What now? The most proven course of action is cognitive behavioral therapy for insomnia (CBT-I), or as we like to call it, sleep hygiene on steroids.

CBT-I is a treatment for addressing the anxieties and thoughts that inhibit sleep as well as your thinking about sleep itself; if you're worried about not being able to sleep, those worries can become a self-fulfilling prophecy. CBT-I helps you change that mindset. This type of treatment has a high success rate: It's been shown to be just as effective as sleep medications in the short term and even more effective in the long term. And it's been shown to work specifically for women in perimenopause. In 2016, researchers led by a team at the University of Washington in Seattle tested the efficacy of telephone-based CBT-I on women between the ages of forty to sixty-five. They divided the women into two groups, with one receiving CBT-I therapy sessions, and the other receiving generalized menopause education sessions. Over the course of eight weeks, the women had six sessions, each lasting about twenty-two minutes. At the end of the eight weeks, the CBT-I group had better-quality sleep, less wakefulness, and an easier time falling asleep than the menopause education group. The number of hot flashes they reported remained the same in each group, but the CBT-I women scored lower on the Hot Flash Related Daily Interference Scale, a tool that measures the impact of hot flashes on daily activities. In other words, they were still flashing, but it seemed to bother them less.

We recommend that our patients start with a CBT-I app called CBTi Coach. It was developed by the United States Department of Veterans Affairs (mobile.va.gov/app/insomnia-coach), so it's free and easy to access, making it a great first step. The app helps you track your sleep for a few weeks, then provides personalized tips on how to reduce wakefulness. If you're not having success with the app, then you might want to seek additional help from a professional CBT-I therapist, which generally involves four to eight sessions. The Perelman School of Medicine at the University of Pennsylvania maintains a directory of international providers (cbti.directory) who specialize in the technique. Most university medical centers with sleep centers can also help you find a CBT-I therapist.

When You Need Something More

So you've done the sleep hygiene, tried CBT-I, and you're still finding sleep elusive. What's next? One option is pharmaceuticals. As we said earlier, CBT-I has better long-term results than sleep medications like Ambien (zolpidem), Lunesta (eszopiclone), and Desyrel (trazodone) and over-the-counter pills like Benadryl (diphenhydramine), which is why we always recommend it first. But sleeping pills can be really helpful in the short term, as long as you're taking steps (like CBT-I) that will actually solve the problem and not just disguise it the way pills do. We sometimes prescribe sleeping aids for a patient just to help her get started with addressing a sleep problem or if nothing else is working, but we advise taking them no longer than a month. This worked well for one patient, Jamie. She had had insomnia for years but had mostly gotten it under control until perimenopause hit. All of a sudden, the wheels came off the bus. She couldn't get to sleep; she couldn't stay asleep. She was operating on two hours of sleep a night. And CBT-I wasn't working for her, at least not through the app. Rebecca prescribed Ambien just to get her back in the habit of sleeping until she could work on some other solutions, such as trying CBT-I again (this time with a therapist, instead of just the app).

Another reason pharmaceuticals don't work well as a long-term solution (and sometimes aren't a good choice even in the short term) is that they can alter your sleep stages. They might put you to sleep for eight hours, but if you haven't cycled through all the important stages, you might still wake up feeling unrefreshed or even feeling like a dopey mess the next day. The changes pharmaceuticals make in your patterns of light and deep sleep diminish the important restorative effects of different stages, and that lack of quality sleep will add up over time. Some research has even shown that long-term use of a class of drugs called anticholinergics, which includes Benadryl and some other antihistamines, is linked to a higher risk of dementia. Your doctor can help you figure out which sleep aid is best for you, taking into account your history and the underlying causes, but for all these reasons, we recommend only using it as a stopgap while pursuing more long-term solutions.

There are some nonprescription options, but it's important not to rely on them for long periods of time either. Some of our patients have asked us about using cannabidiol (CBD) products like gummies, and the truth is, we just don't know. Because cannabis has been a federally prohibited drug for so long, it is not well studied. Does it disrupt sleep patterns? Is it a good short-term solution? Is it harmful in the long term? The answers are not in yet.

Melatonin supplements come up in patient consultations, too. This is another over-the-counter option that we don't know enough about. Some researchers have found that 3 mg of melatonin improves sleep in perimenopausal women, but it's important to note that more melatonin is not better. Bumping it up to, say, 5 mg won't get you an extra two hours' sleep. And, while this is something you might want to try, it's best to think of it as a short-term solution since it's uncertain whether long-term supplementation makes natural production of the hormone go down.

While we don't recommend taking sleeping aids long-term, there are some pharmaceutical treatments that can be helpful during perimenopause specifically. One of the first we try for patients is micronized progesterone. As we've mentioned, progesterone is soothing to the brain. Progesterone increases dopamine and GABA, and these can help your brain calm down, relax, and thus help prevent waking. While micronized progesterone is only FDA-approved for fertility enhancement and to counter estrogen in hormone therapy, it can, at your physician's discretion, be prescribed "off-label," and many women find it to be incredibly helpful in deepening sleep. (One caveat: There is a small subset of women whose brains, in fact, are agitated, not soothed by progesterone, but there's no way to know before trying it.)

Another way to benefit from the calming effects of hormones is birth control pills (which may also help treat other perimenopause symptoms, as discussed elsewhere in part 2 and in part 3). Birth control pills contain progestogens, a category of compounds that bind to the progesterone receptor. There are two kinds of progestogens: progesterone and progestins, both of which are used in contraceptives. Pills that contain progestins won't help with sleep directly, but they do suppress ovulation and help reduce hormonal variability, which can ease anxiety, and in turn help with sleep.

The best treatment path also depends on the root cause of your difficulty sleeping. Micronized progesterone can help with anxiety and general regulation of circadian rhythms during perimenopause, but if your problem is night sweats, it's not going to be as helpful (although some studies suggest higher than usual doses may be beneficial). If temperature regulation is keeping you awake, estrogen might be a better solution. Estrogen helps regulate body temperature during the night, keeping it low and steady. We've seen patients respond beautifully to estrogen, reporting that they're sleeping much better and feel more rested and energetic the next day.

If you or your doctor think you might benefit from both progesterone and estrogen, Menopausal Hormonal Therapy (MHT) can be a great option. MHT is used to counteract a number of different perimenopausal symptoms (see chapter 13 for a full discussion), but some patients find it particularly helpful for sleep. Amy had a patient, Carla, a forty-six-year-old whose main perimenopausal complaint was sleep disturbance. Carla had always been a good sleeper, but for the past year she'd started to experience the typical 2 to 4 a.m. wake-up we see in many perimenopause patients. She'd been to a sleep specialist, who prescribed trazodone, but even with the sleeping pill, at best she was getting only three hours of sleep a night. At that first consultation, she had only slept four or five days in the last month, and, to be frank, she looked it, with huge circles under her eyes. Amy was actually worried that Carla's sleep disruption was going to be too far gone for even menopausal hormone therapy. But she and Carla agreed that Carla would do a trial of MHT. It was a huge success. At Carla's three-month follow-up, she was a completely different person. She was bright and vibrant. She was joyful. She said the hormones gave her her life back. She felt like herself.

This is a great example of one of the key takeaways from this book and the perimenopausal transition in general: Hormones don't have the same effect on everyone. The solution that sent your older sister into deep slumber unfortunately might not prevent you from tossing and turning all night. But that's why we recommend keeping an open mind. Even if it takes some stops and starts, work with your doctor to find the solution that suits you best.

Beating the Heat

There's one other treatment we recommend if your sleep struggles are due to hot flashes—and it's not a pill or any kind of medical intervention. It's called the Chilipad, and it can be a huge help for those who are finding temperature to be a particular challenge—for Rebecca it was a lifesaver. Because she had breast cancer (more on this in chapter 16), she was not a candidate for the hormones that might have alleviated her night sweats. Instead, she found the Chilipad, which is a cooling device that lies on top of the mattress and is attached to a cube that sends cool water through the pad. The temperature of the water can be adjusted to whatever works for you—some people like it cooler than others. This or other similar products can be a great solution, especially if you and the person you sleep with have temperature incompatibility issues.

Which brings us to another potential solution: the sleep divorce, otherwise known as sleeping in separate bedrooms (if you're lucky enough to have an extra room with a bed). If your partner is not another perimenopausal woman, they may need a warmer room than you, and this can become a bone of contention. Once, during her perimenopausal stretch, Rebecca's husband came in and said, "It's 40 degrees in here! You have every window open and it's 20 degrees outside." "Yes," she'd replied. "Isn't it awesome?" He went and slept in the other room during the winter and she stayed, perfectly happy, in the 40-degree room.

Sometimes you just have to adjust for a couple of years. You can still have sex in the same bed and it doesn't mean you don't love each other. But sleep is important. And this can head off some other problems, too, like the partner whose schedule is opposite yours and is always crashing around the bedroom waking you up, or, as people begin to do at this age, is snoring loudly enough to exacerbate the insomnia you already have. Sleeping separately can help both of you get a good night's rest.

5

Mood Swings

Like PMS on Steroids

Once, during perimenopause, I became so angry at my ten-year-old daughter that I took her piggy bank and threw it to the ground, shattering it into pieces. Why would I do such a thing?

—NOW-MENOPAUSAL WOMAN LOOKING BACK

At some point a few years ago, Rebecca realized that she had heard an unusual but similar story from three different patients: They'd developed a fear of bridges. None of the three could drive over the bridges themselves, and when someone else was driving, they had to close their eyes. This might not seem like much of a problem, but bridges are just about unavoidable in the Seattle area where the patients live, so it was a real handicap. And their fear seemed to come out of nowhere.

Even though the world at large still thinks (if they think about it at all) that perimenopause is all night sweats and heavy periods, it can wreak havoc on your mental health as well. Like puberty and pregnancy, the hormonal variations of perimenopause can throw you for a loop. Emotional and psychological symptoms like irrational phobias and other heightened types of anxiety, feelings of anger, panic, depression, prolonged irritability, sullenness, weepiness, and moods that swing as wildly as a jazz piano metronome, can all be directly related to perimenopause.

Research has shown that, during the menopausal transition years, there's a fourfold increase in a woman's risk of depressive symptoms and a two-and-a-half-fold increase in the diagnosis of major depressive disorder. In 2020, the National Center for Health Statistics reported that the rate of antidepressant use for women doubles after age forty, from 10 to 20 percent. (While the study was released in the fateful first year of the COVID pandemic, the data was from 2015–2018 and unrelated to the epidemic.) Anxiety rates rise during the perimenopausal years, too. In the general population, anxiety disorders affect 1.9 to 5 percent of people in midlife. Among forty-five- to fifty-five-year-olds, the diagnosis among women is double that of men.

Like all perimenopausal symptoms, this emotional volatility will affect some people more than others. You may escape mood shifts almost entirely, while other women you know will experience them severely, and others will be somewhere in the middle. We don't know for sure if the hormonal fluctuations of perimenopause are the cause of these rises in depression and anxiety. There are undoubtedly a lot of social and emotional factors women have to deal with in midlife that also drive mood. As usual, it's likely a combination of both, but whatever is at the root of how you're feeling, these mental health symptoms should not be swept under the rug. And it's important to remember that a lot of the mood-related symptoms of perimenopause abate once you hit menopause, especially if you're one of the people who experience more severe changes. It won't be like this forever!

What It Feels Like and Why

Before perimenopause, you might have found it fairly easy to recover from challenging moments. Your teenager would talk back to you, and while you might not be thrilled, you'd shrug it off. If a colleague criticized your work, you'd talk through it, get clarity, and move on. When your spouse forgot about your tax returns, you'd call him out and joke about the IRS coming after you. But now in these moments, you stew and obsess, get irrationally angry, or catastrophize. You scream back at your teenager. (*What kind of kid am I raising?*) You give your colleague the cold shoulder. (*She is out to get me!*) You worry that your spouse's laxity is going to make you miss the deadline (*I know it's weeks away, but...*). Once you hit perimenopause, something going wrong can send you into a tailspin, and it's a horrible way to feel.

Mood swings are one of the factors that make perimenopause feel like that "second puberty" we talked about in chapter 2. Perhaps you not-so-fondly remember the days when, as if your developing body wasn't enough to contend with, you had to deal with emotional highs and lows. If you've erased those memories from your mind, maybe you're seeing it in your own children, where the smallest incidents take on earth-shattering proportions and grumpiness rules the day. There are a lot of the same biological dynamics at work in puberty and perimenopause, the big one being unpredictability. The brain does not respond well to unpredictability, and during perimenopause, hormones are anything but predictable.

During an average menstrual cycle, as we outlined in chapter 2, your brain, or more specifically, your pituitary gland, releases follicle-stimulating hormone (FSH), which prompts the follicles in the ovaries to ready eggs for potential fertilization. Once you hit perimenopause, a lot of these eggs are subpar; they don't develop properly and don't send the correct signals back to the brain. So the brain continues to signal and signal the ovaries to keep trying to produce a quality egg. (This is pretty similar to what happens during puberty, except that in puberty the body struggles to create viable eggs because it's so new to the game and hasn't perfected it yet, which also creates inconsistency.)

Before you reach perimenopause, your hormones are typically produced in a regular cycle, with relatively low spikes of estrogen and progesterone at different times of the month. After ovulation, the levels of both hormones gently drop off, causing the mood shifts you may have experienced during PMS. In perimenopause, this neat little cycle goes out the window. There are times when estrogen and progesterone are produced in very high amounts and then in very low amounts, and that affects the brain in ways that can feel like falling off an emotional precipice. In a premenopausal cycle, PMS mood shifts are caused by the drop in estrogen and progesterone recounted above. But the descent isn't as precipitous—more Acapulco cliff-diver jump than Everest descent—so while you may feel off, it probably won't seem as dramatic. And if it does feel dramatic—all PMS symptoms, just like perimenopausal symptoms, vary among individuals—it won't last as long because your cycle will restart on schedule and bathe your brain in hormones again. In perimenopause, however, these hormones can drop even more drastically, and the volatility can really impact your emotions.

How exactly do reproductive hormones like estrogen and progesterone influence your brain and mood? It hasn't been studied very well and consequently we don't have a great understanding of what's going on. But we do know a few things (some of which we outlined in the previous chapter on sleep). Both estrogen and progesterone (as well as testosterone) affect the brain's neurotransmitters—little messengers that enable cells to "speak" to each other through a combination of electrical and chemical signals. In the brain, neurotransmitters help specific brain cells (neurons) to communicate, and that communication is important for optimal brain function, including keeping your mood elevated and relatively steady. When the communication among certain brain cells breaks down, you can become susceptible to depression and anxiety and their offshoots like phobias, anger, irritability, and despair.

Estrogen, specifically, promotes the production of the neurotransmitter serotonin. Serotonin is sometimes referred to as a "feel-good chemical" for its positive effect on mood. Estrogen also prevents the neurons that synthesize serotonin from reabsorbing the chemical (called reuptake), so it stays in the brain longer. Selective serotonin reuptake inhibitors (SSRIs) are a category of antidepressants that work in much the same way that estrogen does to keep serotonin circulating in the brain, which makes it, and us, happy (among other things). Estrogen and progesterone together have a similar effect on dopamine, another feel-good neurotransmitter that enhances feelings of satisfaction and pleasure.

Progesterone influences mood in a few ways, too, but primarily by interacting with the GABA (gamma-aminobutyric acid) system, which we mentioned briefly in the last chapter. GABA is a particular type of neurotransmitter that actually blocks exchanges between neurons. While communication between neurons is important, too much communication can be a bad thing. GABA plays a critical role in quenching overexcitability in specific brain cells, helping to control anxiety, fear, and stress. Progesterone heightens GABA's effects, which promotes feelings of calm in most people.

As with all perimenopausal symptoms, you may escape mood shifts almost entirely, while other women you know will experience them severely, and others will be somewhere in the middle. There are also a range of mood-related symptoms, and they run the gamut from merely bothersome, like irritability, to serious, like depression. No one likes to feel cranky or overly emotional, but those feelings tend to be easier to live with and less worrisome than anxiety and depression. As physicians, we take these symptoms very seriously and you should, too.

Anxiety in Overdrive

Your level of anxiety during perimenopause may depend on how well your brain adapts to the hormonal fluctuations. Some people's brains simply adjust better than others. Others may find themselves so consumed with worry that they develop general anxiety disorder (GAD), a catchall term for various manifestations of feelings of worry, dread, and fear. Anxiety can show up in a lot of ways, including feeling constantly on edge, having trouble concentrating, developing headaches and/or stomachaches, or finding it hard to sleep. But you might also be unable to stop worrying, become restless, and find it difficult to relax.

Beyond GAD, some studies have shown that perimenopausal women are more vulnerable to one type of anxiety disorder in particular: panic attacks. Typically, panic attacks are an amalgamation of symptoms, which can include a pounding or racing heartbeat, sweating, shaking, feeling like you can't breathe, dizziness, and chest pain. Other times, panic attack symptoms might be less dramatic (but still confusing). When she was forty-five, one patient, Natalie, found herself having heart palpitations for extended periods of time for no apparent reason. A faithful exerciser, she had always had good cardiac reports and usually had a calm demeanor. She also was an older full-time working mom with a young child at home, who was struggling in the relationship with her own mom. And she was deep into perimenopause. But it never occurred to her that perimenopause had anything to do with the racing of her heart. Her family physician never brought it up either but did send her for an EKG and stress test. Both showed that Natalie's heart was fine, and everyone chalked it up to stress.

We're glad Natalie got her heart checked out—it's always important to be sure there's not an underlying issue—but if Natalie had come to us first, we might have dug a little deeper after the cardiac checkup to see if other symptoms she was experiencing pointed to perimenopause, instead of just everyday stresses. We would have talked to her about how hormonal fluctuations during this time of life can trigger heart palpitations by ramping up anxiety. In her case, it was both—stress at home plus disarray in her ovaries led to some scary (but ultimately harmless) experiences. And that's the case for a lot of women.

You might be more likely to develop disabling bouts of anxiety during perimenopause if you've had prior episodes, depression, or post-traumatic stress disorder (PTSD). It's also not uncommon to feel anxiety symptoms most intensely in the morning. Cortisol, the stress hormone that precipitates that fluttery fight-or-flight feeling, is at its highest level in the body upon waking. Add to that the fact that low estrogen increases cortisol, and you may wake up feeling awash in anxious thoughts. We'll tell you how to help mitigate these difficult feelings later on, but first, we want to address the other big emotional risk during this time: depression.

More Than Just Feeling Sad

Around the world, about half of women between the ages of forty and sixty-four report having symptoms of depression during the menopausal transition. And there is evidence to suggest that there's some cause and effect. In 2006, researchers in the Department of Psychiatry at Harvard Medical School published findings from a study of women ages thirty-six to forty-five who'd never suffered from depression before. What they found was that those women who began perimenopause during the study's seventy-two-month duration were twice as likely to develop depression as those women who had not entered perimenopause.

This doesn't necessarily mean you're destined to experience depression, or anxiety for that matter. But it's important to be aware that perimenopause-related depression does exist so that if you do start experiencing some of the hallmarks of the condition (see "Signs of Depression Mood Disorder" on page 80), you don't dismiss them—or let others dismiss them—as just a "hormonal thing" and not seek help. There are also a few factors that can increase your likelihood of developing depression. The Harvard Medical School study and other investigations have found that women experiencing hot flashes have a greater incidence of depression. Why there's an association between the two is unclear. It could be ascribed to what the researchers call the domino theory: hot flashes (which we'll explore in chapter 11) disrupt your sleep; then your lack of sleep can contribute to developing depressive symptoms. It's also possible that the same hormonal inconsistencies that trigger hot flashes may also inhibit the circulation of serotonin in the brain, thereby also triggering depression.

If you've had depression before entering perimenopause, that also puts you at a higher risk for more of the same. Women who've previously had depression are thirteen times more likely to experience it during perimenopause and eight times more likely to have it after menopause. Another risk factor for depression during perimenopause is postpartum depression. In both cases, progesterone levels dip precipitously (the same thing that happens in a less intense way during PMS!), depriving the brain of the soothing effects that keep us on an even keel. We also feel there are similarities in how both postpartum depression and perimenopause have been regarded by the medical community. For a long time, PPD was dismissed as "baby blues," and women suffering were simply dismissed or worse, shamed for their symptoms. Now it's well recognized that the huge drop in progesterone after childbirth can cause a major depressive disorder. It's a very real, physiologically driven phenomenon that requires support and treatment.

Similarly, the mood swings of perimenopause have historically been brushed off by physicians, even though they can be debilitating and put women at risk of suicidal ideation. According to the Centers for Disease Control, the age range of women associated with highest risk for suicide is forty-five to sixty-four: prime menopausal-transition years. (For men, who have a much higher rate of suicide than women, the rate is highest for those aged seventy-five and older.) Some of what we know about the link between perimenopause and suicidal ideation comes from a 2009 European epidemiological study of close to nine thousand women and men. The people participating in the study were from six Western European countries and ranged in age from eighteen to fifty-eight years and older. Researchers found that perimenopausal women were seven times more likely to think about ending their lives than men of all ages and women in other phases of life (including menopause).

The study had some limitations—among them, the perimenopausal cohort was much smaller than the number of people in other groups—but it does echo what some other investigators have found. For instance, in a 2023 study published by researchers in Japan, perimenopausal women reported more thoughts of self-harm than women who hadn't started the transition yet. Since the study began before the women reached their perimenopause years, the researchers were also able to tease out whether there was anything associated with preventing thoughts of suicide. There was: Those women who indicated they had social support were less likely to have suicidal ideation.

We don't share this information to scare you, but to demonstrate how seriously we take the mood changes that can occur during this time, and you should, too. Don't hesitate to ask for emotional support from loved ones during this time. If at any point you experience thoughts of suicide, don't just rely on those around you; please seek professional help immediately. In the United States, the Suicide and Crisis Lifeline is 988, and you can text them as well as call them on the phone.

The good news is that for many women, this level of emotional upheaval is limited to the menopausal transition. For the most part, depression that comes on during this time generally recedes during and after menopause (though people who suffered from depression before the menopausal transition may be an exception). When statisticians at the University of Pennsylvania Perelman School of Medicine crunched the numbers in 2016 as part of the Penn Ovarian Aging Study, they found that the risk of depression was very low within two years of a woman's final menstrual period. This was true for both Black and white women (no other races were included in this particular study). So if you're struggling, know that this is likely temporary. And in the meantime, there are many treatment options available, which we'll discuss in the next section.

SIGNS OF DEPRESSION MOOD DISORDER

You don't have to have a clinical diagnosis of depression to justify seeking help. If depressive feelings are interfering with your life, that's enough. Don't suffer in silence. And especially don't suffer in silence if you're experiencing any of the signs below.

- Feelings of hopelessness and/or worthlessness

- No interest or pleasure in the activities you usually love

- Deep fatigue, lack of energy

- Difficulty concentrating, remembering, or making decisions

- Significant changes in sleep or appetite

- Aches or pains that do not have a clear physical cause

- Thoughts of death or suicide or suicide attempts

What You Can Do About It

If you find yourself struggling with emotional and mental health issues, no matter what's causing them, no matter how severe, there's no shame in asking for help. And this is especially true if the symptoms are affecting the quality of your life. By that we mean if your state of mind is causing trouble in your relationships with friends, family, colleagues, or your partner, if it makes you less able to function well day-to-day, or if it changes your communication style in ways that make you less likely to be listened to, we strongly recommend talking to your doctor about what's going on to see what they might be able to do about it.

As we've just recounted, there's a hormonal component to all this emotional upheaval, but it's also important to assess what else is going on. The feelings that may lead you to smash a piggy bank, write a scathing letter, yell at a spouse, or feel so down in the dumps you stop leaving the house can be multifactorial. Sometimes, it's the fact that after forty years of living, you have simply had enough of the layers upon layers of responsibility, expectations, and just trying to keep a hundred balls in the air as most women do. Women have a reputation for being "too emotional," but in our observation, we women get very good at controlling our emotions. And after a while, they build up. So yes, maybe the hormonal shifts are contributing to outbursts or feeling blue, but they could also be a sign that you need a break or need to shake things up.

THE GRAY DIVORCE PHENOMENON

While the divorce rate for younger people has fallen, the rate for middle-aged and older adults has risen to a not-trivial 36 percent, or 1 in 3, according to a 2022 study published by sociologists at Bowling Green State University. Divorce in these later life stages is colloquially called "gray divorce," though you don't have to have gray hair to pursue divorce later in life.

Do perimenopause and menopause figure into gray divorce? They might, though research is not conclusive. In 2022, a survey conducted by the Family Law Menopause Project and Newson Health Research and Education in the UK found that seven in ten (73 percent of one thousand) women blamed the menopausal transition for the dissolution of their marriage. Sixty-seven percent said it increased domestic abuse and arguments. Additionally, 80 percent said perimenopause/menopause symptoms put a strain on family life. Other surveys agree that the menopausal transition can put a strain on partners, but still others suggest that perimenopause and menopause are not major factors in divorce among middle-aged and older couples.

From our vantage point, it's likely that both situations can be true. When a marriage or longtime partnership ends, it's rare that there isn't a confluence of factors involved. We both have had many perimenopausal and menopausal patients come in and tell us that their relationship, which they've been in twenty or so years, has gone to hell and they're sure that their symptoms are the cause. What relationship wouldn't be affected by a decreased desire to have sex, anger and resentment toward a partner, loss of confidence due to physical changes, sleeplessness, and a partner's lack of understanding of or empathy for your symptoms?

And yet, here you are in midlife, with years of experience and acquired wisdom. Maybe you're just seeing more clearly now. Certainly, if you find yourself inching toward a gray divorce during these middle years, it's worth making a genuine evaluation of whether your symptoms are playing a role. But we're also proponents of following your gut. You're the best judge of how you feel in your relationship. How big or small a role are your symptoms playing in its changing tenor? Maybe it really is time to break up. But maybe it's also worth putting on the brakes to see where you are when your symptoms ebb, either naturally or through some kind of treatment. We counsel patients to think of it like having surgery. They tell you never to sign any papers until twenty-four hours after you come out from under anesthesia, and you should probably think of these menopausal transition years the same way. If possible, don't sign anything without considering what role symptoms are having in your situation.

There are many available treatments that can be very helpful in treating the mental health symptoms of perimenopause. Here's an inventory of your options, which range from minimally invasive to more serious alternatives.

➤ **Movement:** The number one recommendation we give our patients struggling with mood issues is to get moving. Go outside, move your body, and get some natural light for at least fifteen minutes a day, more if you have the time. You don't have to speed walk, or carry a backpack, or wear a weighted vest, walk up hills, or do anything overly strenuous. You just need to walk for a while and let the light hit you. There's considerable evidence that natural light improves symptoms of depression and encourages a better night's sleep (see chapter 4). We find that getting in the habit of walking outdoors every day really helps patients with perimenopausal symptoms. We do it ourselves. The combination of moving and being outdoors is one of the reasons people feel better when they go on vacation.

➤ **Meditation:** It's been shown many times over that meditation can help worry and sadness abate, and researchers in China have found that it can specifically help during perimenopause. In a study published in 2020, 121 women ages forty-five to sixty engaged in an eight-week mindfulness-based stress reduction therapy that utilized techniques popularized by Jon Kabat-Zinn. The women attended two hour-long classes a week during which they went through muscle relaxation and breathing exercises, guided meditation, tension release, and a little stretching. They were also asked to continue the techniques at home on their own. After the eight weeks were up, the women had lower scores in depression, anxiety, and sleep disturbances. And the more often they practiced on their own—some practiced frequently, others sometimes, and some not at all—the lower their scores in these areas were.

➤ **Social connection:** As you might remember from the earlier mention of a Japan study about suicide ideation, the women less likely to contemplate dire acts were those who had substantial social support. It's widely accepted that connection with others reduces everything from chronic to serious illnesses while improving stress management and overall mental well-being. (Social connections help people live longer, too.) So this is no time to be shy: Seek out friends and family. It will help you, too, if you can connect with people you can talk to about your perimenopausal symptoms: You need and deserve support. If you live within proximity of female relatives or have friends who have gone through or are currently going through the same transition, they can be important resources to help weather this particular part of the perimenopausal storm.

➤ **Therapy:** If your symptoms are severe, or even if you wouldn't categorize them as severe but they're disrupting your life, we recommend seeing a therapist. In some areas, including the Seattle and San Francisco Bay areas, where we practice, we're fortunate enough to know psychologists who specialize in issues like perimenopause and menopause. That's where we send our patients. Unfortunately, this isn't an option for everyone, and even seeing a practitioner who specializes in the menopausal transition via telehealth isn't always possible. But a good therapist can definitely help alleviate symptoms, even if they don't specialize. Ask your family physician or ob-gyn for a recommendation. Therapy is an especially good idea if you find that a past trauma is resurfacing. About 50 percent of all women have experienced some sort of trauma, sexual or otherwise, and it's not at all unusual for an issue to resurface when brain chemistry changes. We'll talk more about this in chapter 7.

➤ **Cognitive Behavioral Therapy (CBT):** Some research shows that CBT may be a particularly effective type of therapy for women in perimenopause. In the chapter on sleep, we talked about CBT-I, which is a special kind of CBT aimed specifically at treating insomnia, but CBT in general can be helpful in addressing many other issues. CBT is based on the idea that changing your thought patterns can help with issues like depression and anxiety, as well as alcohol and even marital problems. CBT therapy teaches coping skills, how to recognize distortions in your thinking, and usually some kind of relaxation technique. In one study, 50 percent of women in all stages of the menopausal transition—perimenopausal, menopausal, postmenopausal—achieved about 50 percent improvement from depressive symptoms through sixteen weeks of CBT. A good portion of the perimenopausal women (26 percent) attained complete relief.

➤ **Hormonal therapies:** There's good data to suggest that, during perimenopause, hormonal medications and antidepressants can be equally effective in improving mood, especially if you are someone who is encountering depression or anxiety for the first time in perimenopause, or who has a history of PMS or PPD. The question of which hormonal medication might help—birth control, menopausal hormonal therapy (MHT), or something else—is a more difficult one. If you're still having a regular (or irregular but it's still happening) menstrual cycle, and your hormone levels are seesawing with attempted ovulation, starting low-dose MHT may take the edge off. And that may be all you need to blunt the dips. But MHT doesn't actually stop your body from trying to ovulate, so your body will still be making all these excess hormones that can mess with your brain's feel-good chemicals.

On the other hand, if you're having huge mood swings or significant anxiety, especially if you're in the early stage of perimenopause, a better course of action may be to take hormonal birth control pills that suppress ovulation. Sometimes it's not entirely clear which is the best pathway, so your doctor might try one approach and, if it doesn't work, then try another. It's a bit like figuring out what contraception method is best—the solutions aren't one-size-fits-all, so it may take some fine-tuning and even require a couple of months to get it right. The good news is that there are a lot of hormone-based options out there to help you cope with the symptoms. As long as you and your doctor continue to communicate about your symptoms and how the medications are working, you can keep making adjustments until you figure out the best option for you. In our clinics, we always make sure to tell patients up front what we think is going to work first and ask them to keep in close communication so we can determine if it is in fact helping or we need to go in another direction. (We menopause-transition specialists don't give up easily!) That's something you can do when working with your healthcare provider, too: If a medication isn't helping, don't think of it as the end of the road. Say so and ask to talk about other possible remedies.

We'll go over more of the specifics of MHT and contraception in chapters 13 and 14, but we wanted to be sure to flag them here, since they can be a great treatment option for mental health concerns that pop up during perimenopause.

> **Antidepressants and anti-anxiety drugs:** Antidepressants are a common tool doctors use to help patients of all ages who are struggling with different mental health issues. In perimenopausal women, antidepressants have been proven to help with depression, anxiety, and other mood-related symptoms, as well as symptoms you might not expect, like hot flashes. When we have patients who've successfully used a particular antidepressant at other times in their lives, we'll likely suggest that they try that drug again during perimenopause. Generally, though, we'll try a hormonal option first (birth control or MHT) to treat the underlying causes, and if

that doesn't work as well as we want it to, we'll usually recommend layering in an antidepressant.

There are a lot of different antidepressants out there, and in order to choose the right one, your doctor will need to factor in what other symptoms you're experiencing and what's bothering you most beyond mood issues. If you're struggling to sleep, an antidepressant that's stimulating may do more harm than good. If your libido has dropped steeply, you may not want to end up taking one of the antidepressants that extinguish the sex drive. Some antidepressants can also make it difficult to achieve orgasm during sex. If you've gained weight, you likely don't want one that may make you gain more.

Depending on your symptoms, your doctor may recommend an anti-anxiety drug like an anxiolytic instead of an antidepressant. There are a lot of options, and if you don't like the effects of one drug, there are many others your doctor could try. As with hormonal medication, there's an art to getting it right and it can take some time, but you can help your doctor do a better job by talking about *all* your symptoms, even ones that feel a little embarrassing or scary to bring up.

➤ **Combination therapy:** Some of the people who have the most difficult time during perimenopause are those who already had a history of severe PMS. Rebecca had a patient, a woman named Liz, who was a high-powered executive at a bank. For many years, she'd been coping, and coping fairly well, with premenstrual dysphoric disorder (PMDD). But when she hit perimenopause, the extra hormonal volatility made her PMDD so much worse that she became completely debilitated and suicidal for two weeks of every month. As a result, she ended up losing her job and going on disability. Liz and Rebecca agreed on a plan of action using a combination of oral contraceptives and antidepressants. But Liz's depression and suicidal ideations didn't significantly improve right away; it took time and patience for the combined medications to work.

What we can learn from patients like these is that, whether due to someone's particular physiology or other unidentifiable factors—sometimes these things are a mystery—it can be particularly difficult for some people to cope with changing hormones. For Liz, it necessitated staying on the medication for three years until she naturally hit menopause and was able to go off the pills. She never did go back to her high-stress career—she chose a less hectic job instead—but she did return to a fully functional life.

6

Vagina Trouble

Dryness and Other Discomforts

My vagina is shut down for business—at this point, intercourse is basically like having sex with a sandpaper condom.

—FORTY-SIX-YEAR-OLD PERIMENOPAUSAL PATIENT

So, we talked about your period, we talked about sleep, we talked about how you're feeling. Any problems with sex? Any other issues you want to talk about?" asked Amy as she wrapped up a consultation with Kate, a forty-five-year-old patient. "Nope, nope, everything is fine," said Kate, and got up to leave. But then as soon as she put her hand on the door handle, she turned and said, "Oh, well, you know, having sex really hurts now." Like a journalist who doesn't reveal the most important part of a story until well into the fifth paragraph, Kate had buried the lede.

There's a lot about perimenopause and menopause that goes unspoken, but probably nothing is less talked about than vagina trouble. Many patients are reluctant to talk about any changes related to their vagina, and understandably, and some physicians even skip over discussing it for fear of making their patients uncomfortable. But your vaginal health is important, and changes during this time can cause problems you may never have expected to your vagina and nearby organs like the bladder, which is why we always make a point of directly asking patients about their sex lives and any changes they may be experiencing.

Symptoms involving the vagina are more likely to happen in menopause—50 to 70 percent of women in menopause have some type of vaginal symptoms—but they can start in perimenopause. Common symptoms can include pain during sex, irritation, itching, and burning, and a change in smell and discharge can come along with perimenopause. One day, you may not think about your vagina at all, the next it suddenly feels like the Sahara Desert, or you're peeing every time you sneeze. Or maybe you're just noticing little changes and unsure whether to bring them up. We're here to explain some of the common symptoms and their causes and empower you to talk to your doctor about them.

What It Feels Like and Why

The combination of hormonal swings and aging tissues can affect the vagina and the vulva in a variety of ways. The most common symptom is vaginal dryness, which is a natural response to the reduction in estrogen in the body during menopause. You may or may not experience this during perimenopause as well—the hormonal volatility during this time makes it hard to predict what symptoms will hit you and which you'll avoid—but if you do, it can be useful to know that it will likely continue (and that there are treatments to help deal with it!). Many other perimenopausal symptoms get better over time, but this is one that is almost guaranteed to stick around.

What's going on, physically, that creates so many unexpected changes during this period? Let's start with a bit of anatomy. While we know the term "vagina" is often colloquially used for the whole area, we're going to use the technical language so we can get specific about what might be happening. We'll use the term "vulva" to refer to the genital area on the outside of your body, including the two sets of genital "lips" (the labia majora and labia minora), the opening to the vagina, the clitoris, and the urethral opening (where urine comes out). When we use "vagina" in this chapter, we specifically mean the canal that connects your vulva to your uterus.

The tissues of the vagina and vulva are a many-layered thing. They have several "basement" layers, and the top layers are thick, folded, and elastic, with many blood vessels that aid in lubrication. As you age, and estrogen drops, the architecture of these tissues begins to change. Elastin and collagen, the proteins that give tissue its elasticity and structure, diminish, so the layers become much thinner and less pliable. (This happens to the rest of your skin, too, which is why we get wrinkles and start to see other kinds of skin changes as we age.) As these tissues start to thin and the lubricating blood vessels recede, the tissues become very flat rather than pillowy and folded as they are during premenopause. The diminished blood flow and change in tissue composition even changes the color of your vagina. The appearance of a premenopausal vagina is bubblegum pink and sort of ruffled, while a postmenopausal vagina is light pink, almost white, and smooth. The changing architecture of the tissues makes it harder for them to stretch. This reduction in elasticity, along with dryness associated with lower estrogen, makes the vagina prone to little abrasions from friction, which in turn can make penetrative sex very painful. Some women even feel discomfort as they go about daily living.

Perimenopause can also create changes in the bacterial ecosystem of the vagina. We have bacteria everywhere—including our skin, mouths, and (as we're reminded in every yogurt commercial) our guts. Vaginas are no different. If everything is going well, we live in symbiotic harmony with our bacteria. Like many relationships that exist in nature, it's mutually beneficial. (Think of the little oxpecker birds that pick ticks and fleas off rhinos; food for the birds, comfort for the rhinos.) In the gut, bacteria help us metabolize different foods and drugs. In the vagina, lactobacilli digest some of the shredded skin cells and generate an acid that affects the pH, making the vagina inhospitable to yeast and creating a happy environment conducive to sperm motility.

During perimenopause, the constant shifting of hormones disrupts the pH of the vaginal microbiome and sometimes creates problems. The vagina becomes less acidic and therefore less friendly to the good bacteria. It also allows other types of bacteria to creep in, and that can result in something called bacterial vaginosis, a condition that can make you itch and/or burn and have a fishy-smelling discharge. It's easy to confuse this for a yeast infection, and the anti-itch components of over-the-counter yeast infection treatments can help, but they won't cure it. Often, your body can recover from bacterial vaginosis on its own, as the microbiome shifts, but it's always a good idea to check in with your doctor or a clinic to make sure you get the right treatment for whatever's going on. There is emerging data that the bacteria of bacterial vaginosis can be passed between partners, so if it keeps happening, you might get more relief if your sexual partner is treated as well.

WHAT DOES CLEAN MEAN?

Like vaginal and vulvar health, vaginal hygiene is an important topic that is often given short shrift, but it's important to understand what "clean" means for the vagina and how to keep it that way. First, avoid washing your vulva with soap. Soaps have detergents, which strip the oils from skin, and that can add to the dryness you may already be experiencing. Water is generally enough; when it's healthy, and the bacteria are all in harmony, the vagina is self-cleaning. If you feel you need more, use a mild face wash with no detergents added. And, while we don't mean to put a damper on a current trend, we recommend you refrain from removing the hair from your vulva. The hair is there for a reason. It keeps the good bacteria and dryness-defying skin oils in the neighborhood. And don't douche either. It flushes the good bacteria out and lets the bad bacteria get in.

There's societal pressure to have a pristine, odorless vulva/vagina, but the truth is, the vagina always has a smell. It may change as you go through the menopausal transition, so it may be different than what you're used to. But most likely it's not a sign that your vagina is in trouble. If it seems terminally "unclean" and you're worried about an odor, a discharge, or anything else, talk to your physician about it.

Other conditions that are sometimes confused with yeast infections are autoimmune disorders of the vagina. One in particular, called lichen sclerosus, can occur, then get worse during this midlife time period. Lichen sclerosus causes your own body to attack the tissues of the vulva. For reasons unknown, the body seems to think these tissues are foreign and sends an army of immune cells to strike out at them. It can occur on other parts of the body as well, but when it's in the genital area—we're not going to pull any punches here—the itching can be really bad. Some patients have even reported being woken from sleep because the itching is so powerful. (Another perimenopausal symptom affecting your rest!) The attack on the tissues also leaves a white film over the skin and collapses the architecture of the vulva. The tissue becomes so fragile that it is easily torn, developing tiny fissures, which are like paper cuts. The vaginal opening shrinks, too, so sex can be very painful. Women who have this condition can be asymptomatic for years until a dip in estrogen triggers symptoms.

Not everyone will experience these conditions, but they're more common during the menopausal transition than other times in your life. We want you to know about them so if signs point in their direction, you can be ready to talk to your doctor about what's going on. Whatever your symptoms are, you and your doctor want to stay on top of them because certain conditions (like lichen sclerosus) can raise your risk of vulvar cancers during this time. And we just want to make sure you get treatment for whatever might be happening. Many women we know believe you only have to visit your gynecologist for a Pap smear every five years, but we encourage you to go every year, especially during this time of life. Various conditions can crop up, and regular checkups will catch them.

Bladder Issues

While it's not part of the vulva or vagina, the bladder experiences some changes during this time as well, and it can be affected by the changes occurring next door in the vaginal area. Just like the skin of your vagina and vulva, the walls of the bladder also get thinner and less elastic during this time. And the weakening of vulvar tissues around the urethra opening can make it easier for bacteria to get into the tube (the urethra) that leads to the bladder. Changes in the vaginal microbiome may allow more pathogenic bacteria in the area, which can lead to bladder infections and urinary tract infections (UTIs).

As the walls of the bladder become thinner and less pliable, urinary leakage becomes more common as well. Whatever you call it——incontinence, an overactive bladder—it's guaranteed to piss you off (pun intended). There can be any number of triggers. Coughing. Sneezing. Laughing. Running. Opening your front door. (There's even a name for that one: Key in Lock Syndrome, which refers to having a strong urge to pee and/or leakage the minute you put the key in the door because of the association your brain makes with the opportunity to use the bathroom.) Besides all the other matters we recounted, with age the bladder is also subject to loss of muscle, just like other parts of the body. Typically when you cough or sneeze, the sphincter muscle that controls the flow through the urethra tightens up. But as that sphincter slackens with muscle loss and lack of elasticity, it stops preventing leakage as well as it used to.

What You Can Do About It

The first thing we want to do is strongly advise you against using any folk remedies for vulvar pain and itching. We completely understand that sometimes symptoms can feel unbearable, but things like capsaicin cream, hydrogen peroxide, boric acid, mentholated rubs, or any of the other home remedies we've heard people say they've tried can be severe irritants and can harm the delicate skin of your vagina and vulva. There are better solutions available that will result in long-term relief and, crucially, won't harm your body.

When symptoms are caused by a bacterial imbalance, we often begin with antibiotics, just to get rid of the "bad" bacteria and help enable the "good" bacteria to thrive. We also add in localized, vaginal estrogen, which resets the pH to the right level, thickens the tissues, and makes them more supple. Vaginal estrogen can be a good solution for many problems. It comes in a few different forms—suppository gel capsule, tablet, ring, and cream—and it's inserted into the vagina. It's localized, meaning that, if used properly, it doesn't course through any other part of the body. This means that it won't help with other symptoms you may be experiencing, like hot flashes (there are other medications we use for that), but it can be enormously helpful for vaginal issues, including vaginal dryness. We generally recommend the suppository over the cream partly because it allows for a controlled dose, ensuring that very little estrogen, if any, is absorbed through the vaginal walls (it is also a bit less messy). Estrogen cream is a little harder to dose, and we need to be aware of its potential effect on other bodily systems, but it can be really helpful for improving the external tissues of the vulva.

There are also solutions that don't contain any hormones. Vaginal moisturizers are an over-the-counter solution for dryness that doesn't involve hormones and can be useful for relieving symptoms and making sex less painful, depending on the level of dryness you're experiencing. We recommend vaginal and vulvar moisturizers that contain hyaluronic acid, a molecule that retains water. And keep it simple. Skip the ones that have herbs and scents and/or twenty thousand ingredients in them. The more ingredients, the more likely a product is to be irritating. Moisturizers are not used with intercourse (they're not lubricants) but can do a nice job of adding moisture to the tissue so that intercourse is less painful. For intercourse, we recommend looking for an over-the-counter lubricant. There are two kinds of lubricant on the market: water-based and silicone-based. Water-based lubricants get absorbed into the tissues, which is great for moisturizing them but can make intercourse sticky. Silicone keeps the vagina slippery the whole time but is not suitable for use with silicone toys or latex condoms, so it's important to know what you'll be using it for before you buy.

While we recommend buying a lubricant intended for sexual use, you may have lubricant alternatives already in your kitchen cabinet. In a pinch, olive oil is an effective natural lubricant for the vulva and vagina (but don't use extra-virgin olive oil, which is more acidic than its counterpart). Virgin coconut oil can be used as well, but keep in mind that oil of any kind can degrade latex and should not be used with latex condoms. You can still get pregnant, and STIs can happen at any age, so practicing safe sex is just as important during perimenopause as it is at other times in your life.

If you have conditions that are making your vagina and vulva itch, sting, or burn, try using a benign barrier ointment like Aquaphor or a diaper cream to alleviate the discomfort before you're able to see your doctor. For lichen sclerosus, you'll need something stronger, so your doctor will likely prescribe a steroid ointment to turn down the immune response, accompanied by localized vaginal estrogen to counter the thinning of the vulva from the steroid. Remember that certain conditions like lichen sclerosus and other similar autoimmune diseases are chronic, so you need to use the medication indefinitely, even if you feel like your symptoms have abated.

Some of our patients have asked us about "vaginal rejuvenation," an umbrella term for procedures said to improve vaginal tightness, elasticity, and dryness. There are some surgical remedies, but the most popular treatments are those done with energy-based systems like lasers and radio-frequency ablation devices (essentially microwaves that destroy cells and tissue). While these remedies were originally designed to tighten vaginal tissues for increased sexual pleasure, some of the makers turned around and marketed them to women in menopause, claiming that they could bring back the normal architecture of the vagina and increase lubrication.

None of the vaginal rejuvenation procedures have great studies supporting their use for treating changes due to perimenopause and menopause. The makers of a laser-based system called the MonaLisa Touch found that a number of women thought that they got better after treatment and had less pain with sex and better lubrication and elasticity. The company also did a couple of very tiny studies where they actually did biopsies or tested the pH of the vagina and showed positive changes. However, they didn't get FDA approval for those indications, because the studies weren't randomized. What they did get was "FDA clearance," which essentially means it's not gonna kill you. *Your treatment is regarded as safe, but we [the FDA] are not saying it actually does anything. You can sell this thing, but we're not approving it to treat X, Y, or Z.* After this, the makers of these types of devices for vaginal rejuvenation extensively marketed them to doctors. They hit the marketing really hard but then stopped doing studies on the devices' effectiveness.

And not all the devices were the same. Some were actually just skin lasers for facial rejuvenation augmented with a vaginal probe. The companies said, "Hey, you can stick this in the vagina, too." And as treatment with these devices became more popular—they began appearing not just in doctors' offices but in medi-spas—we started to see some complications when they were operated by untrained hands. Not a lot of them, because these devices are pretty low-power, but problems like vaginal burns and abnormal contractions of the tissues that narrowed the vagina too much began to be reported. More than hurting people, they just weren't doing anything, and women were spending a lot of money to get mostly nothing done. Some women found that it helped with urge incontinence, the strong desire to pee and leakage, and there is some evidence to suggest lasers may help with lichen sclerosus. But if you think logically about some of the other promises, how can something both tighten the vagina and create more elasticity? They are diametrically opposed. You could do one or the other perhaps, but vaginal rejuvenation was usually marketed as doing both.

In 2020, researchers from an array of institutions (Stanford, Brown, the Cleveland Clinic among them) published results from a randomized controlled trial called the VeLVET Trial, which compared treatment with a CO_2 laser (the MonaLisa Touch) to treatment with vaginal estrogen. The trial was stopped midway by the FDA because a particular exemption for using the device in studies was not obtained first. The group, however, was able to report the early results, which showed that estrogen and the laser were essentially comparable in terms of improving sexual function and urinary incontinence symptoms. It wasn't, however, a slam dunk since the study was halted after six months. More recently, a European randomized trial looked at the CO_2 laser compared to a sham laser. In both sets of patients, the probes were inserted and noises were made so nobody (neither the doctors nor the patients) knew whether they were getting a real laser treatment. In that study, both groups of patients had the same outcomes, which basically means that the laser is unlikely to be doing anything. We're probably seeing a placebo effect.

So what is the bottom line here? Some women really swear by these laser treatments and have seen improvements in incontinence and lichen sclerosus. Rebecca was an early adopter of the vaginal rejuvenation laser procedure for perimenopausal and menopausal symptoms because it showed promise. But as more data came in, she couldn't in good conscience continue to offer the treatment (which is not covered by insurance). The research proving its effectiveness just wasn't panning out.

We always recommend vaginal estrogen first. Still, it should be noted that some women don't want to use any estrogen at all, and some patients also report that using a combination of the two, laser and localized estrogen, worked better for them than either alone. If this is a therapy you want to try, it isn't likely to hurt you—if you're in the hands of someone well trained, and who can counsel you on other options (like vaginal estrogen). See a gynecologist or a urogynecologist. Don't let someone at a medi-spa near your vagina.

Make Your Bladder Better

Our first recommendation whenever someone is experiencing leakage is pelvic floor physical therapy. The pelvic floor is the group of muscles around your bladder, uterus, and rectum that work together to support those organs. When we talk about strengthening the muscles in this area, most people think about Kegels. Kegels are pelvic floor exercises that strengthen the muscles that hold the bladder and other organs in place, and they can help with urinary (and fecal) incontinence. But they don't help with other problems that cause leakage. We're advocates of pelvic floor therapy because there may be some areas of the pelvic floor muscles that are overly lax, but other areas that are overly tight. Sometimes the bladder leaks because your muscles are already in such a heightened state of tension that they can't tense any more. If you raise your arm and make a muscle by squeezing your biceps, then try to squeeze it some more, you'll see that it doesn't go much further. That's the same thing that can go on with the opening of the bladder.

Physical therapy (PT) helps you get everything back into balance so you can have all the muscles work together synergistically to control the flow of urine. A really good therapist will be able to tell which muscles are overworking and which are underworking and help you get them into the same state. Achieving this goal can also help with painful sex. The pelvic floor can be like your shoulder muscles when you're tense—clenched—and you can imagine what trying to have intercourse when the muscles around the vagina are closed for business will be like: It's going to hurt. PT can help relax this area and mitigate any spasming or cramping you might experience.

Another treatment we use for urinary incontinence and bladder infections is, maybe surprisingly, vaginal estrogen. By changing the pH and, subsequently, the bacterial makeup of the genitals and by plumping up the tissues in the vulva, vaginal estrogen makes it less likely that any bad bacteria will climb into the urethra. There are also other prescription medications specifically for overactive bladder (where you feel you have to pee every fifteen minutes). These work by decreasing the signaling in the bladder so it doesn't react to running water or the key in the front door. For very recalcitrant cases, there are tiny devices that teach the nerves to stop firing and triggering the urge to pee. They're actually implanted in a nerve near the ankle, which when stimulated sends signals to the bladder. Your doctor can help you figure out what might be the best solution for you.

While changes to the vaginal area can be stressful, we hope it's a relief to learn that there are many remedies available to help you cope with any issues you're having. Whether you'll *want* to have sex, even if it feels good, is another topic entirely. We'll explore libido in the next chapter.

7

Disappearing Libido

Not Tonight, I Have Perimenopause

I have a great relationship with my partner. I want to have sex with them. I just cannot do it right now because I feel so terrible.

—FORTY-FIVE-YEAR-OLD PERIMENOPAUSAL WOMAN

We hear a lot about "dad jokes" these days; it's become a whole subgenre of comedy. Well, here's some mom humor for you: What do moms agree is the sexiest thing on the internet right now? Pedro Pascal in gladiator garb? Idris Elba's knowing grin? Harry Styles's tattooed torso? How about men emptying the dishwasher. Vacuuming the house. Taking care of the kids. That's what passes for mom porn these days.

Even though mom porn is a joke (though, like most jokes, based on truth), this is a roundabout way of saying that women's sexual desire is not straightforward. What turns us on is complex. So when sexual desire begins to mellow and perhaps even evaporates, there is usually a tangled web of factors involved in its decline.

Contrary to what popular culture suggests and the onus society puts upon us, not everyone of all ages is having sex all the time. It's completely normal for libido to wax and wane, but the hormonal wackiness of perimenopause, on top of other experiences of aging, can make women's sex drives plummet.

If you're comfortable with a lower sex drive, that's great! But if your sex drive has declined during this time and that bothers you, there are a lot of ways to raise your libido and get excited about sex again. The medical phrase for when there's a mismatch between how much sex you want and how much sex you *want* to want is "sexual dysfunction." "Dysfunction" makes it sound like there's something wrong with you if you don't want to have sex. That's not true. You're allowed to not want to have sex. But if your lack of desire causes you distress—meaning you wish it was different or your partner wishes it was different—that's when it's called sexual dysfunction.

Sexual desire, in many women (and men as well), has been shown to decline in midlife and beyond, but sexual dysfunction among women of all ages is actually quite high, with an estimated 43 percent prevalence in the general population. This number is even higher in cancer survivors, ranging from 50 to 90 percent. But the menopausal transition does accelerate change. One study, the Melbourne Women's Midlife Health Project, showed that the percentage of perimenopausal and menopausal women with sexual dysfunction rose from 42 to 88 percent over a nine-year menopausal transition period. What's going on here? And what can be done to help?

What It Feels Like and Why

Sophie and her husband, Will, had a quip they'd use when things were about to get intimate. "Sex," they'd say to their dog, King, and he'd get the message, jumping off the bed as they laughed. But when Sophie began experiencing perimenopausal symptoms in earnest, King's spot on the bed was nearly always secure. Sophie just wasn't very interested in having sex.

Probably the most common kind of sexual dysfunction we see is when you just aren't very interested in sex. It doesn't mean that you don't love your partner or that you're not attracted to them. It's just that you're not in the mood. Ever. Or mostly never. Or you may be okay once it's started, but you never initiate sex anymore. Another sign that something has changed is that, whether you have a regular partner or not, you rarely have a sexually tinged thought anymore—so strange because you used to be the woman who spent her twenties and thirties imagining erotic couplings with various people who crossed her path. And if you do have sex, you may just not enjoy it as much. Maybe you find little pleasure in the act, are less likely to have an orgasm and, when you do, it's not the fireworks you remember.

Is it hormones? Researchers have long wondered if there is any relationship between sexual desire and hormonal fluctuations across the menstrual cycle. At first they tried to discover the answer to that question by noting how often heterosexual women had intercourse during various times of the month. Those studies concluded that the menstrual cycle didn't affect sexual habits and thus, presumably, sexual desire. But then someone came up with the brilliant notion (we say this facetiously) that women often have sex when they don't especially desire it and that they often *avoid* having sex when they're most likely to become pregnant. So just looking at when women have sex didn't really answer the question.

Back at the drawing board, other researchers tried a different tack: They asked women to note when they had feelings of sexual desire regardless of whether they had intimate relations with anyone at the time. Some researchers also looked at the relationship between masturbation and the menstrual cycle and whether lesbians, whose sexual timing didn't involve worries about pregnancy, seemed to be hornier at particular times of the month. What all these studies found was that there's a correlation between ovulation and increased sexual interest, peaking when estrogen levels are high and right before the egg gets sent down the chute. And, of course, this makes evolutionary sense: Sexual desire ups the odds of intercourse when it's most likely to help perpetuate the species.

So, yes, at certain times of the month, if you're having regular menstrual cycles, there's an estrogen factor in spontaneous desire. It follows then that, in perimenopause, when the cycle and hormones get wonky, that type of out-of-the-blue arousal may go out the window and explain some loss of libido. But there's another kind of desire, called "responsive" desire, which many women experience more often than—sometimes to the exclusion of—spontaneous desire. Responsive desire is a sexually charged reaction to touch and other forms of intimacy. Maybe in the past you weren't likely to think to initiate but would find yourself responding (the operative word) with desire to someone else's initiation. This kind of desire can also go out the window with perimenopause and is harder to measure in relation to hormones.

If estrogen seems correlated with more spontaneous desire, what about testosterone, which is often touted as a libido enhancer? There's little evidence to suggest that a woman's natural production of testosterone is a central player in her sex drive. If it was, we might expect libido to *increase* during perimenopause and menopause since testosterone becomes more bioavailable as estrogen declines, and its production doesn't change significantly during the menopausal transition. Nonetheless, supplementary testosterone can boost libido. Doses that approximate what you produce naturally—which is what we consider safe—won't turbocharge your sex drive, but they will give it a little lift. (More on testosterone later in this chapter.) While it's clear that there's some hormonal influence on sex drive, there are just too many factors to pinpoint any specific cause of waning libido in perimenopause.

If your desire for sex has taken a hit as you've moved into perimenopause, there could be several reasons, some obvious, some less so. For instance, pretty incontrovertible is the fact that vaginal dryness usually affects sexual activity. If sex hurts, you're not likely to want it. If you have had sexual trauma in the past, pain can also bring it up again to the point where your body says, "I'm not accommodating this anymore."

Many of the other common symptoms of perimenopause can also dampen desire. Poor sleep (too tired for sex), hot flashes (too sweaty for sex), mood swings (too irritable for sex), achy joints (too sore for sex) . . . you get the picture. Perimenopause can also make you feel lousy, and hardly anyone wants to have sex when they don't feel good. Sexual desire can be tied up with self-esteem, too, and the physical changes to your body during perimenopause can really impact your confidence. The good news is that when we treat the common symptoms and patients sleep better, feel less anxious, and aren't dealing with vaginal symptoms, many people find that their lust returns.

The stress of midlife can also just make sex hard to prioritize. If your desire is mostly the responsive type, it might be difficult to dedicate energy and attention to the kinds of tenderness and touch necessary to build up to desire. And if you're not having sex, and there is a mismatch in the relationship, it can make the tension around sex even more stressful, putting a huge damper on your arousal. When you don't want to have sex, you're less likely to spontaneously touch your partner, hold hands, kiss them, or do anything else that might give them the mistaken impression that you're in the mood. When you withdraw in this way, you lose the intimacy and closeness that drives responsive desire so then you *really* never feel like having sex.

Whether your lost libido is due to physical changes or psychological ones, there are a lot of ways to rekindle passion in both long-term and new relationships. In fact, studies show that "New Relationship Energy" (a term psychologists like to use) brings about a return of spontaneous lust even in perimenopausal and postmenopausal women. But regardless of your situation, there are many ways to restore your arousal and enjoy sex well into your later years.

Arousal Disorders

Often, the typical drop in libido experienced by perimenopausal women is treatable using perimenopause- and menopause-specific therapies. "But there are also sexual arousal disorders that can affect women of any age and that have both physical and psychological underpinnings," says Leah Millheiser, MD, a female sexual medicine and menopause expert at the Palo Alto Medical Foundation. These disorders have multiple causes, among them depression, certain medical conditions (such as multiple sclerosis, diabetes, peripheral vascular disease), or medications (including combined hormonal contraception and SSRI antidepressants). The menopausal transition, too, can be a factor. "During and after the menopausal transition," says Dr. Millheiser, "these arousal disorders become more prevalent due to declining estrogen levels."

Arousal disorders typically result in less vaginal engorgement (blood flow) during sexual activity, and that decreases sensation and lubrication, and can also make it difficult to achieve orgasm. This constellation of symptoms adds up to something known as genitourinary syndrome of menopause (GSM), a progressive condition that impacts up to 84 percent of perimenopausal and postmenopausal women. Some women going through the menopausal transition can also be affected by persistent genital arousal disorder (PGAD), a less-well-understood condition that's associated with unwanted, intrusive sensations of genital arousal in the absence of sexual desire. It likely affects anywhere from 0.6 to 3 percent of the population.

We'll offer a number of suggestions in this chapter that we've seen work for our perimenopausal patients, but if you think your difficulties with arousal might be more than just the combination of midlife distractions and hormonal fluctuations, it might be a good idea to get evaluated by someone who specializes in sexual medicine. There are many ways to treat sexual arousal disorders, including with sex therapy; relationship therapy; off-label use of Viagra, Wellbutrin, and other medications; topical estrogen; and even devices like vibrators. Some of these are particularly useful during perimenopause, but a sexual medicine practitioner will be able to identify the best solution for your specific condition.

What You Can Do About It

Before you get started on the fixes, it may be useful to assess how much of a problem your lack of sexual desire is in your life. As we said earlier, loss of sexual desire isn't a problem unless you feel it is. For some couples, the mismatch of sexual interest can be a huge bone of contention, so if your relationship is important to you—or simply because sex is important to you whether you're part of a couple or not—the issue deserves your attention. We'd like to note, though, that sexual disinterest can go both ways. We have patients who come in and say, "My husband doesn't want to have sex anymore" or "He has erection issues, and I feel the loss." So it happens on both sides.

When it's on your side, first consider that loss of libido is typically multifactorial and may require treating it from a variety of perspectives. The first step is to fix the pain if pain is indeed a factor. About 50 percent of women we see experience pain during sex due to vaginal changes (as outlined in chapter 6). Eliminating pain can go a long way in helping your sex drive. You may not yearn for sex the way you used to, but you'll definitely enjoy it a hell of a lot more, which is the first step to wanting it more often. Next, consider what you may be able to do to fix other perimenopausal symptoms, like managing stress or resolving sleep issues. Sleep divorce, which we talked about in chapter 4, can sometimes be just the thing couples need to reinvigorate their sex lives.

If other symptoms are not at play or vanquishing them doesn't make you any more amorous than before, consider the big C in sexual relations: not carnal knowledge, not clitoris, but Communication. Sex can be a difficult thing to address in a relationship, but talking about it can lead to working together on strategies that will help you regain sexual intimacy. One of those strategies is thinking of sex as a habit that needs to be reinstated. Thinking about sex as something routine isn't very erotic, but consider that, as our colleague Ashley Fuller, MD, likes to say, sex is kind of like going to the gym. Almost nobody wants to get out of bed and go to the gym in the morning, but you set the alarm, wake up, say to yourself, "It's good for me so I'm going to go," put on your sports bra and leggings, and get yourself there. And while you're at the gym, and your energy kicks in, you think, "Oh, yeah, this feels great." After it's done, you're so glad you did it. Sex can be like that, too. Sometimes you just have to figure out how to make it a regular thing.

We're big fans of the psychologist and author Laurie B. Mintz, PhD, and one of the recommendations she makes in her book *A Tired Woman's Guide to Passionate Sex* is to schedule sex. It might seem unsexy, but many people find it really helps introduce sexual energy back into their relationships. A patient of Rebecca's, Christine, made it work by scheduling sex with her husband on Saturday mornings. Kids away at college, not a work day, what could stop them? The plan had some unexpected beneficial side effects as well. Knowing that there was a time for lovemaking in the books, Christine felt freer to touch, kiss, and be physically close to her husband at other times without the fear that she would have to slam the door on sex, because they were going to have sex—it was just going to be on Saturday. Eventually, the renewed intimacy became less rote, more natural, and made sticking to the schedule unnecessary.

It's also worth considering whether your relationship is working well aside from sex. Maybe it's a difficult time for you and your partner outside of perimenopause. As we noted in chapter 5, gray divorce has become increasingly common as women find that their relationships aren't working anymore. If you find that the trouble is bigger than just perimenopause throwing things out of whack, it's worth considering couples' counseling, separation, or a change to your relationship structure depending on what you want from your partnership.

In fact, all of these are issues that can be (and should be) taken up in therapy. You may benefit from couples' therapy, talk therapy, CBT, or even something like sex therapy. Some people are uncertain about what really gives them pleasure—after all, no one really teaches us how to have sex. Good sex therapists can make you feel comfortable talking about things that nobody really likes to talk about with a stranger (let alone their best friend). They get down to the nitty-gritty and they do it without judgment. For help finding a sex therapist, we recommend going to the American Association of Sexuality Educators, Counselors and Therapists (AASECT) website's directory: https://www.aasect .org/referral-directory.

Testosterone for Libido Enhancement

You have now patiently read through advice about scheduling sex and sex therapy, but perhaps what you really want to know is, "Can't I just take testosterone or some other pill and forget about all that other stuff?" We recommend working on the other aspects—especially the communication part—of sexual relations with your partner, because while testosterone can be part of the solution, it's rarely *the* solution. If your partner isn't meeting your emotional or sexual needs and that has pretty much squelched your sexual desire, testosterone can't fix that. Yes, it can heighten your interest in sex, but if you keep the dosage to what we believe are safe levels, it's (as we stated earlier in this chapter) no turbo charge. Ford, not Ferrari. And because of side effects, there are good reasons to be careful with testosterone (see "Why We Object to Testosterone Pellets" on page 111). So if you do want to try it, let us advise you on how to do it safely.

First, it should be noted that there's no FDA-approved testosterone specifically for women on the market in the United States, and there's a story to be told about that. Several studies have shown that testosterone can improve sexual desire in women. In 2019, researchers led by Susan R. Davis, PhD, head of the Monash University Women's Health Research Program, in Melbourne, Australia, did a meta-analysis of thirty-six clinical trials with a total of over eight thousand postmenopausal participants. They found that testosterone, administered by patch, was effective in increasing the number of times women had sex per month as well as their sexual satisfaction.

This would lead you to believe that some company is out there developing a testosterone for women, and you would be right: It's called the AndroFem cream and it was available in Australia, but it has never been available in the United States. While the company behind AndroFem showed evidence that the cream is safe and had no significant side effects (even after extending the study four years to show longer-term efficacy and safety), the FDA still refused to approve it. They believed the boost to sexual function wasn't big enough and that it *might* cause side effects sometime in the future. We have high regard for the FDA, but were puzzled by this decision. (We weren't in the room, but who wants to guess whether or not it was men making the call?) Millions have been spent on ensuring help for men's sexual function (e.g., Viagra, Cialis), but women have not received the same consideration. We don't have a safe, FDA-regulated female-dose testosterone product in the United States.

But this doesn't mean there's no testosterone available to American women. When we (meaning us, Amy and Rebecca) prescribe testosterone, it's usually for women who've tried other means of increasing their sex drive without success. The testosterone we prescribe is in topical forms that the FDA has approved for men (AndroGel and Testim are two brand names), and we prescribe it at about one-tenth the standard dose for men. A man might use 5 milligrams per day; a woman will be prescribed 300 to 500 micrograms. And then we monitor blood testosterone levels to make sure it doesn't get too high. Even at this small dosage, testosterone can help with libido. The effect won't last forever, but it can be a good boost.

However, it's important to be aware of the other effects testosterone can have on the body. If a woman's testosterone gets too high, it can start to have masculinizing effects, so it's important to keep a close eye on blood levels. This is why we're not fans of testosterone pellets, but even topical testosterone can push a woman's testosterone up to masculinizing levels. One patient, Cynthia, came in for a problem unrelated to perimenopause. In the course of two visits, Rebecca noticed that not only was Cynthia's clitoris enlarged but her speaking voice had deepened significantly. She'd gone from a soprano to a tenor. She admitted to taking testosterone—prescribed by someone who wasn't monitoring her levels—but assured Rebecca that it would be okay because everything would go back to normal after she stopped taking the hormone. Rebecca had to be the one to break it to her that those changes would not reverse. If you're going to take testosterone, your levels need to be closely monitored.

WHY WE OBJECT TO TESTOSTERONE PELLETS

Testosterone pellets are tiny, waxy tablets about the size of a grain of rice that are implanted under the skin, usually in the butt. Over the course of three to six months, they gradually release the hormone into the body, then eventually dissolve on their own. Estrogen can also be administered through pellets; some pellets are made up of a mix of hormones. Testosterone pellets often contain what's called supraphysiologic doses of the hormone, meaning that they'll raise testosterone to levels higher than what's normally present in the body. That's the reason pellets (or any large dose of testosterone) can have a stronger influence on libido than a judiciously prescribed FDA-approved topical testosterone. A supraphysiologic dose doesn't replace what your body is missing; it provides an unnatural amount of the hormone, and the lift in libido is a side effect of that extravagant hit.

Pellets are often administered by clinicians at specific hormone clinics, but general gynecologists prescribe them as well, although they're not covered by insurance and can be costly. We like to think that everyone is just trying to help women feel better, but we take issue with the safety of implanting pellets, especially because they're developed by compounding pharmacies out of the purview of the FDA. Clinicians have access to regular forms of hormones that are sold through traditional pharmacies, and, we believe, they should always recommend them as a first line of therapy. If they're not, ask yourself why they're only offering you an option not covered by insurance.

Sometimes the patient's testosterone levels aren't monitored, and that can be problematic, too. Moreover, there's evidence to suggest that pellets have a significantly higher incidence of side effects than menopausal hormone therapy (MHT). Plus, while sometimes advertised as safer and more natural than MHT, the hormones in pellets are no safer or "plant-based" than FDA-regulated versions; in fact, they're the same synthetic hormones, just not regulated in terms of dose and sterility. (And unlike the ones from the pharmacy, they're not covered by insurance.)

High testosterone levels can cause a lot of unwanted side effects. Some are physically harmless but potentially emotionally damaging, like developing masculine features if that's not your goal (and if it is, you still need to be monitoring your testosterone levels in order to avoid more harmful side effects). Excess testosterone can be converted into estrogen in the body, which is bad news if you're diagnosed with breast cancer or another hormonally related cancer, because you can't just take the pellet out. And you don't want estrogen from a pellet or estrogen as a by-product from a testosterone pellet in your system while undergoing treatment. You'd have no choice but to wait out its time-released demise.

The eagerness to feel better, to improve your sex life, especially if it's causing a relationship to deteriorate, is completely understandable. So is the determination of healthcare practitioners to improve their patients' lives. Pellets just aren't the way to do it, especially when so many other—and safer—options are available.

Other Libido Boosters

There are two other medications on the market intended to improve low libido in women. One is called Addyi (flibanserin) and the other is called Vyleesi (bremelanotide). Addyi was originally developed as an antidepressant—it affects serotonin in the brain—and, while it didn't work particularly well in that capacity, it turned out that women who used it had an increase of two to three satisfying sexual encounters per month, which may not sound like a lot, but if you are having *no* satisfying sexual encounters per month, it can make a huge difference. The drug was then approved for treatment of low libido.

Vyleesi also has an interesting development history. It works on the melanocortin receptors in the brain, which affect inhibition. But melanocortin receptors are also in cells responsible for pigmentation of the skin, which is why Vyleesi was created as a self-tanner. It didn't ultimately work to create a Hawaiian glow, but it did seem to improve women's sex lives, so the drug company went in a different direction. While Addyi is a pill you take daily, Vyleesi is an injectable that you administer about forty-five minutes before having sex. It's not great for spontaneous sex, and if you use it often, it can leave a small dark spot at the injection site, but if nothing else has worked, it may be a useful solution. Be aware that these medications are fairly expensive and are not covered by insurance (neither is testosterone).

At the end of the day, prescription remedies work 40 to 50 percent of the time; they're far from a sure thing. But even when they do work, sexual desire usually needs to be nurtured. While quick fixes will wane, if you work on the underlying issues and make time for communication, desire is far more likely to return. Keep in mind, too, that you're in a perfect position to say how much or how little sex is right for you. Don't worry about what everyone is doing on TV (it's fiction!) or what you perceive to be everyone else's very hot sex life (may also be fiction). Figure out what's right for you and your relationship and aim for that.

8

Swelling Waistline

The Midlife Middle

Where did my waist go?

Laurie is a forty-nine-year-old patient of Amy's who lived a healthy lifestyle for decades. With some effort, she had been able to maintain her weight within 5 pounds even into middle age. But then, all of a sudden, things changed. Laurie came to Amy frustrated by the fact that she had gained 10 pounds seemingly overnight (it was actually over a few years, but it didn't feel that way!). And all the weight was collected in her midsection. She wanted to know if there could be a hormonal reason for her otherwise unexplained body composition changes. The answer was yes . . . to an extent.

It can be alarming to gain weight seemingly out of the blue. Maybe *you* haven't altered any of your eating and exercise habits in twenty years, but over that time, your physiology has changed. That's why, when you reach midlife, doing what you've always done before may not keep your weight at its pre-perimenopausal level. Gaining weight during this time is very common, and even if you don't gain weight, you're likely to see some kind of shift in body composition with age.

In most Western cultures, women are conditioned to think that they need to be the same size at every age, even though hardly anyone in their forties and fifties has a carbon copy of the body they had in their twenties. At least not without going to extremely restrictive lengths (or a very good plastic surgeon), and even then, you may never fit into the dress you wore when you got married or the jeans you saved because they once hugged your butt so splendidly. In the same way, we've been inundated with messages that tell us that only thin is healthy. We're learning now that this piece of oft-cited wisdom isn't necessarily true, and the connection between body fat and health is far more nuanced than it might seem.

Even if we know intellectually that the relationship between body size and health is complicated, it can still be difficult to deal with physical changes in a culture that prioritizes youth and thinness. We know from experience that it doesn't feel good to gain weight, and you'll likely want to do something about it. What's important is to find that middle (yes, pun intended) ground, the place where you can feel fit and healthy again without turning your life on its head or devoting your waking hours to the impossible expectation that women's bodies remain ageless. There are changes you can make to meet the perimenopausal pounds head-on, and the first step to managing a shifting waistline is understanding why women in midlife typically gain weight in the first place.

What's Happening and Why

Some reports suggest that women in their forties and fifties gain about 1.5 pounds a year. If that's true for you and you weigh 130 pounds at age forty, by age fifty you may weigh 145. By age sixty, 160 pounds. But of course, we know that bodies are more complex than that, and the amount you gain (because you are likely to gain some weight) could be far more, or it could be far less. One of our patients, Cindy, had kept her weight very strictly in check all her life, just like Laurie. As her body shifted into perimenopause, she noticed that she'd gained four pounds, which sounds like nothing—your body can fluctuate by that much over the course of a day depending on how much water you drink—but for Cindy, this was highly distressing. She began to reduce her calorie consumption to well below recommended levels, and she exercised constantly while training for triathlons. And yet, even though she was still very lean, Cindy had developed a little bulge in her midsection that she couldn't get rid of. Gaining weight in the midsection, specifically, is a classic experience of perimenopause, as Cindy was seeing firsthand.

As women go through the menopausal transition, most of us, even the thinner ones among us, gain not just weight but "central adiposity"—an accumulation of fat in the abdominal area. If you've ever pondered the mystery of your disappearing waist and/or emerging belly, the answer, it turns out, is simply that body composition shifts in midlife. And not for the first time. After puberty, the shape of girls and boys, mostly similar before, begins to diverge due to ascending sex hormones. Girls start to store fat in the breasts and lower body (pelvis, thigh, and butt) regions, creating energy depots that can one day be used to support pregnancy and lactation. Boys, on the other hand, tend to store fat in the upper body. (If you've ever seen a man with a beer belly who seems thin otherwise, you've seen the effects of sex hormones on body composition in action.)

DIFFERENT KINDS OF FAT

Putting on weight in midlife is normal, even if it feels alarming, but it's important to be aware of what that extra weight might mean for your health. The risk of diabetes and cardiovascular disease increases as women go through the menopausal transition, and part of this has always been ascribed to the increase in upper body fat. This isn't something we take lightly—the association between menopause and these conditions is clear—however, we're also beginning to see evidence that belly fat in women is not as harmful as belly fat in men.

Abdominal weight gain results in the addition of two types of fat. The largest percentage gained is subcutaneous fat—fat stored right beneath the skin. The other type of fat we acquire is what's called visceral fat. Visceral fat is found deeper in the belly and surrounds organs like the liver and intestines. It's not always apparent—thin people can have visceral fat, too—and it's the type of fat that's linked to disease risk. In 2021, researchers from Harvard Medical School published findings in the *Journal of the American Heart Association* showing that abdominal fat gain was significantly associated with metabolic diseases (like diabetes, insulin resistance, and non-alcoholic fatty liver disease), heart attack, and stroke in men—but not as much in women. Women are different. This doesn't mean women can't gain visceral fat, or that those with considerable amounts of visceral fat are in the clear, but it can help you breathe a little sigh of relief—the abdominal fat–related health risks for women don't seem to be as dire as we once thought. The study also had another, and perhaps more important takeaway: In women, it's much more important to look at the muscle-to-fat ratio. The women in the study with more muscle had lower risks, no matter what amount of fat sat on top of it—more reasons to introduce strength training into your exercise regime, if you haven't already!

The hormonal roller coaster, the same one that causes mood swings and trouble sleeping, is also behind the shift in fat distribution many women see during this time. When estrogen dips, as it does over the course of the menopausal transition, testosterone availability (not production, just availability) increases and causes the body to start storing more fat in the belly. This seems like a cruel joke, but it can actually be beneficial. There's an evolutionary theory that women store fat in the belly once their reproductive years are through because, if there's a famine, food resources are going to go to the younger people in the community first. That little belly is there to help us weather the bad times.

Another way that extra fat helps is by producing estrogen (specifically E1, or estrone). Abdominal fat cells are not the only other place in the body besides the ovaries where estrogen of any significance is produced, but they do it most efficiently. So when the ovaries' estrogen manufacturing drops off, the body says, "Hey, you're a little low on this; let me help you out. I'm going to give you a life preserver!" (And sometimes it feels and looks like a life preserver!) But even with the abdominal fat cells producing estrogen, the levels of estrogen in the body fall significantly over the course of perimenopause.

Estrogen is also linked to other hormones that affect body weight, and having less estrogen available can impact the levels of these hormones. One hormone affected by a reduction in estrogen is leptin, which is produced in the fat cells and triggers feelings of fullness. Another hormone, ghrelin, is an appetite stimulant made in the stomach. Both of these hormones' levels change with estrogen loss: leptin goes down, ghrelin goes up. Most women we see in our offices claim they're not eating any differently than before, and we have no reason to doubt them. But considering the changes in appetite hormones that occur during the menopausal transition, it's worth asking yourself: Am I really eating the same as I always have? (Or, while we're on the topic of self-observation, are you moving—not just exercising, but moving—as much as you once did? Long days behind a desk, hours sitting in a car commuting and/or shuttling kids to and fro, no time for walks because you have to go over to your parents' house to help them out—it all adds up to less calorie burning.)

As with many other perimenopausal symptoms, there's also an aging component. With the exception of erratic periods and hot flashes, symptoms are hardly ever just a hormonal issue. In the case of weight gain, one of the aging components is muscle (lean tissue) loss. Muscle loss typically begins in your thirties and follows a slow decline of 3 to 5 percent a decade. Accordingly, the ratio of muscle to fat in the body changes, with muscle going down and fat going up. Muscle is a calorie-hungry tissue; the more of it you have, the more calories you burn, so it seems logical that metabolism—the rate at which you burn calories—will decline in step with muscle shrinkage.

Something else you may be up against during this time of life are the waistline-expanding effects of poor sleep. If you're experiencing the midlife wide-awake-and-worried phenomenon we described in chapter 4, this throws an additional risk factor for weight gain into the mix. Just like declining estrogen levels, lack of sleep is linked to higher production of ghrelin (which makes you hungry) and lower production of leptin (which makes you feel less satisfied). That can mess with your appetite and make it harder to put the brakes on eating, even if you've always been very disciplined.

As noted, many women feel like they are still eating as they always have and are still gaining weight despite not consuming an extra morsel. And that can certainly be the case: This is a time when you can gain weight without any alterations in activity or diet. But some perimenopausal women also report feeling like the guardrails have come off their usual calorie-controlled eating, which may be a result of the leptin/ghrelin changes during this time. Beyond how much you eat, these hormones can also influence what you feel like eating—and it's not veggies! Don't be surprised if you crave sweets and starchy foods.

Another weight-gain risk that lack of sleep can set in motion is a metabolism drop. Research shows that getting less than seven hours of shut-eye per night can decrease basal metabolic rate by as much as 400 calories a day. This, combined with loss of muscle, can lead to a general slowing down of your metabolism. In fact, it's long been believed that metabolism slows with age, though some new research out of Duke University suggests that men's and women's metabolism doesn't really slow down significantly until they're in their sixties. Research is still going on in this area, but one thing we do know is that staving off muscle loss through strength training—which we'll talk about later in this chapter—does promote greater calorie burning, as does getting a good night's sleep.

SLEEP AND WEIGHT GAIN

Some of what we know about the impact of poor sleep comes from the Nurses' Health Study in women, ongoing research that began in 1976 and is among the largest investigations into the risk factors for major chronic diseases. In one part of the study, researchers looked at the association between sleep and weight within a sixteen-year time frame. What they found was that women who slept less than five hours a night were 15 percent more likely to become obese over the course of the study than those who slept seven hours. A smaller study, this one published in 2013 by researchers at the University of Colorado, looked at the relationship between sleep and weight by having eight men and women sleep only five hours a night for five days. Another eight men and women slept nine hours per night. Then the two groups switched places. When sleeping for five hours, the people in both groups ended up eating more calories than when they had longer stretches in bed; they even gained a little weight over the course of the five days. Amy's co-residents in her ob-gyn residency called this the food-sleep continuum—the less sleep you have, the more food you eat to help you make it through the day. It explains Amy's twenty-pound weight gain while she worked thirty-six-hour shifts delivering babies for four years straight!

Sleep can also affect weight in another way. Like all hormones, cortisol, known as the fight-or-flight hormone, ebbs and flows throughout the day. At night it drops so you become less alert, allowing you to get sleepy and ease into slumber. In the morning, it rises again, helping you to wake. Poor sleep chronically elevates cortisol, and, since regulating calorie burning is among the several jobs cortisol has in the body, this can further throw the metabolism out of whack. If you think about it, this makes sense from an evolutionary perspective. Our ancestors lived in precarious times, so we evolved to be able to quickly fight or flee predators. As part of this protective system, cortisol helps to slow calorie burning and increase fat storage in the belly so you will have energy for fighting and fleeing readily available.

Of course, unlike the lions that may have pursued your forebears, your modern-day stressors (lack of sleep compounded by midlife worries like too much responsibility at work, relationship drama, kids who won't launch, and so on) require no extra calories and belly fat. But your body's hardwired to give them to you anyway. One of the ironies of all this is that your body is prepped for action, and yet, because you're not sleeping well, you're probably going to be too tired to do anything physically active—another reason perimenopausal insomnia can increase your likelihood of gaining weight. The more tired you are, the less you're going to move and the fewer calories you're going to burn. Plus, who hasn't been so tired they couldn't care less about what they eat? Fatigue is the enemy of healthy habits.

What You Can Do About It

When we talk about weight with our patients, we don't talk about numbers on the scale or pants size. We talk about health. So this is a good time to ask yourself: Is your weight affecting your health? Have you gained so much that you're now prediabetic or diabetic or at a weight that raises your risk of heart disease and cancer? This is something you and your doctor should be tracking. Ask yourself, too: Is your weight making your perimenopausal symptoms worse? We know that women who are heavier have more hot flashes. Weight can exacerbate joint pain and elevate your likelihood of sleep apnea and urinary incontinence. Another potential pitfall of carrying a lot of extra weight in your middle is that the estrogen produced by belly fat can increase the buildup of the lining of your uterus, leading to heavier periods and a greater risk of precancer and cancer of the uterus. On the other hand, if you're frustrated by the extra pounds around your middle, but all your health markers are fine, it may be a sign to try to let go of the body you had in your youth and embrace yourself as you are now.

If you do decide to try to lose weight at this age, first consider that, as with so many other aspects of growing older, the things you did as a younger person may not work now. Your body is different these days and you'll likely need to adjust. Second, be aware that for women in perimenopause and menopause, weight loss tends to be four times slower than in women who are younger, regardless of the diet or method used. It can be a slog. Third, consider that no matter where you are on the perimenopausal weight-gain spectrum, whether you've always struggled with your weight or, until now, have always been the kind of person who can eat whatever they like and never put on extra pounds—reducing the perimenopausal life preserver comes down to three simple things: eating well, exercising in ways that counteract estrogen loss and aging, and getting enough sleep. Yes, sleep. For all the reasons listed earlier, don't leave sleep out of the equation. Rethinking your approach to all three elements affecting body weight may help you shed pounds, but more importantly, each one is key to good health.

We like to use the term "rethinking" because many of you may already be doing things that seem beneficial to your weight and overall well-being. Like Cindy, the triathlete who was down to a minimum number of calories, maybe your routine is quite rigorous. But even

Cindy needed to change. Rebecca's advice to her was to get help with sleep through the cognitive behavioral therapy route we covered in chapter 4. Then she had Cindy work with a nutritionist to improve her eating. Cindy actually needed to eat *more* calories, but higher-quality ones. Her restrictive regimen might have seemed virtuous, but she actually wasn't nourishing her body. Even with all the exercise she was doing, Cindy couldn't prevent muscle cell depletion because she wasn't getting enough nutrients to effectively replace the muscle she was losing.

Eating

When perimenopausal pounds first begin to appear, the temptation is to go on a diet, but we don't recommend this at all. What we recommend instead is eating regularly—breakfast, lunch, and dinner. Fasting, particularly intermittent fasting (going sixteen hours without food, typically from early evening to the next day's afternoon) is a popular weight-control strategy these days, but in our experience, people who are intermittently fasting get so hungry that they binge once the fasting period is through. And they binge on high-calorie, nutrient-poor foods. No one, in other words, is bingeing on carrots. Of course, you can try intermittent fasting. You can try Keto, you can try Paleo, you can try Whole30, you can try the diet everyone in your office is talking about. They may all help you lose weight. But can you stay on them forever? Research and personal observation suggest that almost everyone who goes on a prescribed diet regains what they lost once they stop. Sustainable, slow change wins out over rapid weight loss every time.

What we view as much more helpful is committing to long-term change, not a six-week attempt to blast off the weight. There's no get rich quick scheme for losing perimenopausal pounds. The "secret" is just simple and moderate eating. It's not exciting, not a magic bullet, but effective. Focus on eating regularly, choosing quality foods, and portioning them wisely. We like to recommend the perimenopause plate: fill half your plate with produce (preferably vegetables, but, yeah, some fruit, too), then divide the rest between a moderate serving of protein (which could mean beans or tofu; it doesn't have to be animal protein) and a small serving of complex carbohydrates (like whole grains). It can be as simple as filling 50 percent of your dinner plate with salad or roasted veggies, nestling in a piece of fish or chicken, and adding some brown rice or farro or quinoa. Season and dress them as you like with reasonable amounts of healthy oils like olive and avocado, so they're not bland and don't make you feel like you're being deprived. Perimenopause doesn't have to be the start of steamed veggies for life. Breakfast can be a slice of whole-grain toast topped with an egg, avocado, or nut butter and some chunks of melon, lunch a bowl of leftover brown rice, stir-fried veggies, and shredded roast chicken or tofu.

A critical part of the perimenopause plate is protein. When you shed muscle as part of the natural process of aging, what you're primarily losing is protein, the building blocks of lean tissue. And the body literally hungers to replace it. One theory of appetite and consumption, known as the protein leverage effect, suggests that muscle loss drives increased hunger for protein. But if you don't know that's what your body is craving, you might just eat whatever's available, often snack-type foods with high levels of carbs and fat. When this nutrient-specific hunger is met with additional carbohydrates and fats instead of protein, it results in an overconsumption of calories because those foods aren't as satisfying. Some researchers speculate that increasing protein can reduce and even prevent weight gain during the menopausal transition. Studies have yet to show this specific connection, but we do know that diets with higher protein proportions tend to lead to overall lower calorie intake and greater satiety.

Protein doesn't have to mean meat either. "My personal favorite plant proteins are beans and lentils," says Stasi Kasianchuk, MS, RDN, senior director of lifestyle care at gennev.com. "It's a one-two punch of protein and fiber, maximizing the benefits for muscles, digestion, and heart health. Not to mention that these are cheaper than most animal proteins. I often recommend that patients aim to include beans and/or lentils once a week. Soups, chilis, and curries can be easy ways to incorporate them." Getting adequate dietary protein—20 to 25 grams at each meal—is essential, regardless of where it comes from. And it's especially essential when you're strength training (which we'll discuss in the next section). You need those building blocks in order to get the job done.

Exercise

Strength training (or as it's often referred to, resistance training) is the not-so-secret ingredient to perimenopausal weight-gain prevention. It's critical. Strength training builds muscle, which helps stave off age-related loss of lean tissue and increases the number of calories you burn in daily life. But the benefits don't stop there. Strength training has a positive impact on almost every health factor you want to start thinking about at this time of life. Insulin resistance, for example. As estrogen declines, the body becomes less sensitive to insulin, and as a result cannot properly regulate blood sugar, potentially setting the stage for prediabetes or full-blown type 2 diabetes. Insulin resistance is also associated with heart disease. But there's research to show that strength training improves insulin processing, so when you lift weights, you're not just increasing muscle; you're raising your insulin sensitivity.

If perimenopause has altered your mood, you have another reason to strength train. In 2018, *JAMA Psychiatry* published a meta-analysis of thirty-three clinical trials looking at the mental health outcomes of strength training. The researchers, from the University of Limerick in Ireland with input from scientists from Iowa and Sweden, found that strength training significantly reduced symptoms of depression. Other studies have also found that strength training improves sleep and counters bone loss, two other concerns for perimenopausal women. Of concern to all women: living longer. In a 2022 study of four hundred thousand adults published in the *British Journal of Sports Medicine*, strength training two to three times a week was associated with a 20 percent reduced risk of premature death.

So what do we mean by strength training? Lifting heavy weights is what produces the greatest benefits, "heavy" meaning that you can only do four to six reps and three to five sets before your muscles become too tired (known as failure). If you can work in a routine that hits both your lower and upper body muscles two to three times a week, all the better. Other kinds of resistance activities can be helpful, too. Workouts that use your own body weight as resistance, such as Pilates and yoga and exercises like push-ups, planks, and squats, and using resistance bands can also help you build muscle. You might put on a weighted vest, strap on a backpack, carry weights, or walk up hills to make cardio exercise more of a resistance activity. Just be aware that none of these other forms of resistance are as effective at building muscle as heavy weights. But some strength training is better than no strength training.

If using heavy weights is daunting, consider taking a weight training class or hiring a trainer for a few sessions to initiate you. It doesn't have to be expensive (check your local Y or those clubs that include a few free sessions with membership), and you don't have to sign on for a year of personal training. Just hire someone long enough to give you a routine and teach you proper form. Even thriftier: YouTube. The number of strength-training videos on the internet is immeasurable and most of them are free.

When we bring up strength training to patients, we sometimes get pushback. A lot of women have been told that lifting heavy weights will give them big, bulky muscles. In reality, it's not easy for even young women to put on significant noticeable muscle, and once you've gone through the menopausal transition, your body will not have the capacity to easily build bulky muscles at all. But strength training will help you generate enough lean body mass to help you burn more calories and make you stronger so that everyday activities are easier. With these newly trained muscles, you're not going to need help carrying your groceries or lifting your suitcase into the overhead compartment on a plane.

Incorporating strength training into your life can require some effort and adjustment. Another reason we sometimes get pushback from patients is that they have a certain amount of time during the week slated for exercise and that time is allotted to cardiovascular, get-your-heart-rate-up workouts. They don't want to give up their hill walks with other moms or miss their morning run or workouts on the cardiovascular machines at the gym. And we tell them: Cardio is great, but you need to do both. You can't elliptical-machine your way out of muscle and bone loss.

While strength training is the most important exercise for perimenopausal women because of its impact on overall lean muscle, cardio is incredibly important, too. It ticks off every perimenopausal (and overall health) box: calorie burning for weight control, improved mood, better sleep. Some evidence even suggests it may help with hot flashes. And, as you no doubt know, cardiovascular exercise is associated with a lower risk of many diseases, including those—heart disease, cancer, and diabetes—that become more prevalent in women after menopause. Cardiovascular exercise can even help you live longer. And if you regularly do both cardiovascular exercise and strength training, as we recommend, it increases the odds that you'll have an even longer life. This has been reported in several research papers, including one study by Brigham Young University researchers that found that, while people who did cardiovascular exercise three times a week had a 27 percent lower risk of dying than people who did no exercise, people who did cardiovascular workouts *and* strength training had a 40 percent lower likelihood of dying than non-exercisers. Clearly, it's worth the time and effort to do both.

The Eating-and-Exercise Balance

When trying to lose some of those perimenopausal pounds, think strategically about how you combine diet and exercise. "The physical activity guidelines for Americans are 150 minutes of moderate or 75 minutes of intense physical activity a week. Two sessions of resistance training and some flexibility and balance training is also recommended," notes Kasianchuk. "And the data consistently shows that meeting these criteria lowers the risk of developing chronic disease, including cardiovascular disease, diabetes, and osteoporosis." But shedding pounds and keeping them off usually requires more. "It's likely that closer to 300 minutes or more per week of moderate to vigorous physical activity is needed," says Kasianchuk.

Okay, so you may need to up your exercise. But slashing your calorie intake at the same time may be self-defeating. "I encourage women going through the menopausal transition to think about getting both nourishing *and* adequate calories," says Kasianchuk. "This often runs up against the 'diet culture' narrative to eat less as you exercise more, but our physiology works better when we fuel it optimally to meet the demands of exercise." That means getting a range of macronutrients—carbs, protein, fats—that are rich in vitamins and minerals rather than cutting out one food group or severely restricting your total calorie intake. Remember the perimenopausal plate! Finding the right balance of physical activity and eating well (and enough) will give you the most success of maintaining a healthy weight during perimenopause.

Medications

Menopausal hormone therapy isn't known to cause weight loss—or weight gain. (We'll talk more about what exactly it does and does not do in chapter 13.) MHT may give a small boost to your muscle-building efforts (and by extension help boost your ability to burn calories) through weight training, but it doesn't work alone. When it comes to weight loss, the most common drug people think of is GLP-1. There is a small amount of evidence to suggest that, in obese women, MHT in combination with GLP-1 medications may lead to more weight loss than GLP-1 alone. But even when used alone, GLP-1s, such as Wegovy (sometimes referred to as Ozempic) and Zepbound, have proven to be effective weight loss drugs.

If you're struggling with midlife weight gain and wonder if these drugs, originally created to treat diabetes, are a good solution for you, there are some caveats to be aware of. First, we should say that we always recommend healthy eating and exercise before anything else. Our take on weight-loss medication is that it should only be part of the conversation if you're struggling with obesity. Obesity is a chronic disease. Yes, some of it is lifestyle, some of it is what we have available to eat in this country, but some of it is genetics and no fault of your own, and it needs to be thought of and treated like other diseases.

If you're thinking of treating this chronic disease with medication, you need to settle into the idea that it's a medication you may need to take indefinitely. Taking Wegovy, Zepbound (these are the brand names of semaglutide and tirzepatide, respectively, when used for weight loss), or any of the rest of the "hot" drugs on the market is not a quick way to drop pounds. You can't go on them for a few weeks and then be fine forever after. Once you stop taking these drugs, you gain the weight back. And what we're learning, especially with the newer medications like the GLP-1s, is that not only do you gain the weight back, but it is then harder to lose again because whenever you lose some weight you lower your metabolic rate. What's more, some of what is lost is muscle, so it's vital that anyone taking these drugs also concentrate on building lean body mass at the same time.

Weight-loss drugs work in different ways, and some have multiple effects. One way the GLP-1s work is by slowing the emptying of the stomach so you more or less feel full all the time and are disinclined to eat as often or as much. Another way they work is by quieting "food chatter" in the brain. All that conversation that goes on between the stomach and the head—*Hey, I'm bored, let's eat; oh, that looks good, let's eat*—simply goes away. These drugs were originally designed for diabetics, so they also, through multiple pathways, lower blood sugar, helping to control the disease.

Metformin (brand names include Fortamet and Glumetza) is another drug created for diabetics and can also be an option if you're really struggling to lose weight. It works by helping your cells process both insulin and calories more efficiently. The weight loss is not as dramatic as with some of the other medications, but metformin is very affordable and widely available in generic form. And it's effective, especially in prediabetics.

Also in the pantheon of weight-loss medications is an older weight-loss drug called phentermine, which works as a stimulant, giving you a little more energy, helping you burn more calories, and typically making you eat fewer of them. Another option is the combination of bupropion (an antidepressant with mild stimulant effects) and naltrexone, a medication that's sometimes used in addiction because it changes the reward pathway in the brain. When you put something delicious in your mouth (especially something high in carbs and/or sugar), you get a little hit of the feel-good chemical dopamine in your brain. So what many overeaters are driven by is not true hunger but rather a yearning for that punch of dopamine. Naltrexone works by reducing the dopamine response so that eating doesn't provide the same sort of high that might drive you to do it to excess. It's a great choice for people who tend to be compulsive in their behavior (it's good for quitting smoking, too). Together these medications reduce hunger and cravings, and make you a little perkier.

Any of these pharmaceuticals can be helpful, but we'll repeat the caveats: They aren't a quick fix; you may need to stay on them indefinitely or you'll gain the weight back; you need to focus on lifestyle changes to eat healthfully and exercise (especially strength training to preserve muscle); and they aren't for people who just need to drop five or ten pounds. They are also expensive and often not covered by insurance. When all those factors are considered, the drugs can be a game changer. We have had patients who were always treading water when it came to their weight, then when perimenopause hit, felt as though they'd completely lost control of their body. These patients who've tried medication report that it was like a sea change, not just for their middle but for their mind. All that noise about food, the guilt, and the agonizing over every food decision disappeared. They felt far less depressed and anxious.

There are a number of different strategies you can use to lose weight, but the most important thing is your overall well-being. As women living in a world that values thinness, we cannot help but feel tormented by expectations. According to the media, social and otherwise, we're supposed to look like Cameron Diaz and J.Lo and Halle Berry as we age; yet most of us have no age-defying genes nor full-time personal chef and trainer. *Most of us.* Look around you and you will see that most women have that midlife life preserver. That's how aging works! We're not meant to look twenty until we're ninety. But we can glow with health and fitness at any size and any age. Make obtaining those two attributes your goal.

9

Brain Fog

A Disorganized Mind

Yesterday, I poured hot water into a full canister of
hot chocolate mix instead of into my mug. It was just one of many
weird lapses that are happening to me now. My friend found
her phone in the fridge the other day.

—FORTY-SEVEN-YEAR-OLD PERIMENOPAUSAL WOMAN

As part of our jobs, we often give talks on various aspects of the menopausal transition. And so it was one day at work when a perimenopausal Amy stood in front of her department to expound on a symptom of perimenopause and menopause that is particularly troubling to women: brain fog. "It's like . . . that thing with the . . . whatever," she stumbled along, trying to explain the concept to her colleagues. But she didn't need to explain: She had just demonstrated it beautifully by not being able to remember a word to save her life! Right in the middle of her presentation. Talk about irony.

Brain fog isn't a medical term, but just about every perimenopausal woman knows what it means. It's the sensation that someone's name or the title of a book is hovering around the edges of your brain, but you just can't grasp it. It's that experience of walking into a room and thinking, *I know I came in here for a reason, but I have no clue what that reason is.* It's feeling disorganized, fuzzy, slow. Or maybe, conversely, it's your mind bouncing around wildly like a rubber ball. Some of what happens to the brain during the menopausal transition can be attributed to lack of sleep and depression and/or anxiety, and some of it is actual changes to the brain, as women's brains start to work a little bit differently as we move toward menopause. Differently, but not necessarily worse (though it may feel that way for a while).

No matter what you're feeling, it can be scary. One thing we'd like to make clear before we delve into the details of brain fog is that brain fog and dementia and even the ultimate cognitive decline that typically comes in old age are all *very* different things. All three are worth thinking about, but it's important to bear in mind that they're not the same. Brain fog does not mean you're on the road to dementia nor that you're more likely to develop dementia later in life. You're okay! It may be rough going for a few years. You may have to use some strategies to help you see your way through the fog. But ultimately, the very large majority of you will be fine once you get to the other side.

What Happens and Why

When we talk about brain fog, what we're talking about is the disruption of normal cognition, which the *American Psychological Association Dictionary of Psychology* defines as "all forms of knowing and awareness, such as perceiving, conceiving, remembering, reasoning, judging, imagining, and problem solving." That disruption can play out in myriad ways, with symptoms including:

➤ Forgetfulness
➤ Lack of word and name recall

➤ Trouble concentrating or focusing
➤ Confusion
➤ Losing your train of thought
➤ Mental fatigue
➤ Slow thinking
➤ Difficulty paying attention

It's opening the refrigerator and immediately forgetting why or finding it difficult to concentrate as well as you used to at work. You might forget the name of the movie you saw last night or have to constantly check your calendar to remember your plans for the next day. Luckily, brain fog isn't permanent, though it can be incredibly frustrating.

As estrogen ebbs in the body, your brain's activity and even some of its structures start to transform. These changes are independent of age and directly related to the menopausal transition. And they're a singularly female phenomenon; they don't happen to men. This, however, does not give men the cognitive edge—and it doesn't mean your mental faculties are gone forever. When studies look at the cognitive performance of women both before and after menopause, they find no difference. Hold onto that positive thought while we take you through an explanation of what's going on in your brain.

Even though most of us come through brain fog with our cognitive abilities well intact, there can be several bumpy years because estrogen is so critical to neurological functioning. It's active in every part of the brain. It's connected to how you learn and to how you retain and recall information, including your ability to retain and recall information transmitted in written or spoken words (called verbal learning or verbal memory). It's connected to fine motor skills and the spatial ability that allows you to understand and remember where things are in your environment. It's even connected to how you interpret pain. Estrogen also affects all the systems in the brain that influence mood (as we noted in chapter 5). So when you take estrogen away, some of the areas of the brain become either less active or behave differently, at least for a time.

A study done by Lisa Mosconi, PhD, an associate professor of neuroscience in neurology and radiology at Weill Cornell Medicine (WCM), and the director of the Alzheimer's Prevention Program at WCM/New York-Presbyterian Hospital, showed that the brain goes to great lengths to try to compensate for the loss of estrogen during the menopausal transition. In that study, published in 2024, Mosconi and her colleagues used positron emission tomography (PET) imaging to look at the brains of fifty-four women between the ages of forty and sixty-five. They found that the further along into the menopausal transition a woman was, the more estrogen receptors she had in her brain. This suggests that, rather than just accepting that there's little estrogen to be had, women's brains seemed to be fighting back, trying to grab as much estrogen as possible by creating more places for it to land. For Mosconi and her colleagues, this was surprising. Common wisdom was that as estrogen waned, the brain stopped making receptors for it. But her study showed the opposite. The brain was still looking for estrogen and making structural changes so it could capture every drop. But the additional estrogen receptors were also a sign that lack of estrogen was a problem: The more receptors a woman had, the more she experienced mood and memory issues during the menopausal transition.

In a different study, two researchers, Pauline Maki, PhD, a professor of psychiatry, psychology and obstetrics and gynecology at the University of Illinois College of Medicine, and Nicole Jaff, PhD, an honorary lecturer at the University of the Witwatersrand in Johannesburg, reviewed a raft of studies relating to perimenopausal brain fog and found that the type of cognitive hiccups most widely experienced is those related to verbal learning and memory—in other words, the ability to encode words into your brain and then recall them. There were some lesser effects observed that relate to a slowdown in the processing and understanding of information as well as of the working memory. Working memory refers to the ability to remember and use information in the short term, such as typing the phone number someone just gave you into your contacts app—the power, that is, to take what's in your brain and quickly spit it out. Overall, though, Maki and Jaff found that women's executive functioning—skills like strategic thinking and problem solving—did not suffer through the menopausal transition, and their cognitive function stayed within normal limits.

Just because cognitive function is "within normal limits" doesn't mean it feels that way. If you are used to juggling a ton of different things at once, one little change in your brain's processing capacity might make a monumental difference in your ability to manage everything. Our brains are also strained with information coming at us from the numerous screens we willingly and sometimes unwillingly look at all day, so even small memory lapses or a struggle processing things might feel as though you've pulled one block out of the Jenga tower and now all the blocks are coming down.

Many women find that perimenopause can coincide with attention deficit hyperactivity disorder (ADHD)–type symptoms: trouble focusing, disorganization, problems finishing things, and an inability to multitask, something they may have been so good at just the week before. We've had several patients get diagnosed with ADHD as adults. One patient, Brooke, came to an appointment with the news that, although she had been completely functional before perimenopause, she was now on medication for ADHD. "I was so scattered all the time," she lamented. An ADHD diagnosis might not be solely due to perimenopause—there's more awareness of the disorder and we have better tools to diagnose it now. But hormonal changes can also make it harder to cope with ADHD symptoms that you may have had all along, even if you weren't aware of it. One of the by-products of lowered estrogen levels is a drop in the neurotransmitter dopamine in the brain. ADHD brains are already low in dopamine, so the tumbling level of neurotransmitters can make things worse—and more apparent to you if you're in possession of one of those brains.

Brain fog, whether it's the type that hypes you up or the type that slows you down or some combination of the two, is hardly ever a stand-alone symptom—often, there's something else going on, whether it's depression, lack of sleep, or something else. Brain fog is a classic symptom of depression at any time of life, not just when the mood disorder has been triggered by perimenopause. When patients come in mourning the loss of their focus and memory, we always screen them for depression to make sure that it's not contributing to their muddled thinking.

Lack of sleep can be another contributing factor. If you're having trouble sleeping, it's going to affect your brain power. You don't need a study to tell you that, but just for the record, in one 2021 investigation that Dr. Maki participated in, sleep difficulties were associated with greater verbal learning and memory weakness in perimenopausal women. It's during sleep that we process and fix new memories, so if you aren't doing that effectively, you'll notice what feels like short-term memory loss the next day.

Hot flashes are the third aggravating factor. Research shows that hot flashes are linked to greater lapses in verbal fluency (e.g., *I have my dog's name on the tip of my tongue*) and can bring about changes in the brain, causing minor ischemic (lack of blood flow) events in the hippocampus. This can sound alarming, but scientists haven't seen anything to indicate that this has worrisome long-term effects, and there is evidence that any related structural changes may later reverse themselves.

What You Can Do About It

The best thing about perimenopausal brain fog is that it's temporary. Even if you take no steps to alleviate it, it will, eventually, dissipate.

Some of the suggestions in this chapter can help mitigate the stress of brain fog, but it's worth considering how much it's impacting your daily life. If it's just a nuisance, you might be comfortable waiting it out. If it's affecting your daily functioning in more severe ways, there are a few options to manage it during this time.

Although we know no one who has been forced to leave her job due to brain fog, we have had patients who choose to do so, most times just temporarily. One of them was Cara, a patient of Amy's, who is a tech executive. Cara was in her late forties and still getting periods (so still in perimenopause) when she decided to take a six-month leave of absence from her job. No one was criticizing her work, but the sudden onslaught of forgetfulness and all-around muddled thinking had her feeling like her life was unraveling. She'd gone from doctor to doctor (neurologist, sleep specialist, and more) trying to figure out what was going on. By the time she stepped into Amy's office, Cara was several months into her quest for relief.

For Cara, the solution proved to be menopausal hormone therapy (MHT). When Amy saw her a few weeks later, she was sleeping, her hot flashes were milder and less frequent, and she could focus again. It was a real game changer. MHT, it should be said, is not FDA approved for the treatment of cognitive issues. It's approved for treating hot flashes and improving bone health. It doesn't mean that it doesn't ease a whole lot of other symptoms related to estrogen loss; it just means that no drug company has taken data to the FDA showing that MHT helps with other problems. Some physicians are very stringent and will only prescribe MHT for the symptoms that it's approved for. We don't follow that line of thinking and sometimes do prescribe MHT off-label if the indications are that it will be helpful.

We don't know if MHT directly affects brain fog; the research isn't clear. But we do know that it helps with hot flashes (which, as noted, it's specifically approved for), sleep disruption, depression, and anxiety. When Amy prescribed MHT for Cara, she was hoping that clearing up the other symptoms that so obviously affect how well the brain functions would help clear up Cara's brain fog as well. And, for Cara, it worked. We should note that women on MHT tend to find relief of other perimenopausal symptoms faster than relief from brain fog. Laura, a friend of Amy's, saw several perimenopausal symptoms dissipate in a matter of weeks with MHT, but her brain fog took longer to resolve. Within a few months, though, she was firing on all cylinders.

The key takeaway here isn't necessarily that MHT is the answer to brain fog (though many women find that it helps), but that the best solution is usually to address the other perimenopausal symptoms that contribute to brain fog, like lack of sleep, mood disturbances, and hot flashes. This might mean hormonal therapy, or it might mean pursuing one of the many other treatments available for specific symptoms. Working on sleep through cognitive behavioral therapy, getting a cooling pad to help with night sweats, and looking at whether any problems you're having with anxiety and/or depression warrant medication will also likely help with your mental energy.

So will exercise, both for its ability to promote better sleep and improve mood and because it directly affects the brain. Exercise increases blood flow and nutrients in the brain, and research shows that regular cardiovascular workouts increase the size of the hippocampus, the part of the brain involved in memory and learning. There are studies, too, that show that people who exercise come up with more innovative ideas than people who are sedentary. Sometimes what your brain may need is a calming effect. Exercise can help there as well: It triggers the release of endocannabinoids, molecules we create ourselves that are similar to those in marijuana, and which have a pacifying effect. Just taking a brisk walk every day can be a balm to your brain.

Meditation has a similar brain-calming benefit. It's not something you might immediately think of as a way to improve your cognitive functioning, but, as we've highlighted, anything that helps you diminish stress and anxiety will also help your brain work better. Several studies looking at meditation and cognitive function in both younger and older people have shown a meditation practice has significant benefits. In one study of seventy-three seniors, mean age eighty-one, those who practiced transcendental meditation or mindfulness twice a day for twenty minutes for twelve weeks had improvements in verbal fluency and memory. What's more, in a follow-up three years later, the improvements held.

While not suitable for everyone, if you are one of the people who find that perimenopause uncovers undiagnosed ADHD, specific ADHD medication may help. For those women who've had undiagnosed ADHD and have gotten by with good coping skills until perimenopause hits, medication can lessen distractibility and boost concentration. If you don't have ADHD, however, you're not likely to see much benefit. That's likely because ADHD is a fundamental brain-wiring problem while what happens in perimenopause is more related to the brain being deprived of one of its prime messengers: estrogen. While ADHD medication may be able to help with focus, it's not necessarily going to help with other brain fog symptoms, such as problems with working memory or remembering words.

Like a lot of phenomena that arise in midlife, brain fog may just be your new normal for a time. Depending how much it is (or is not) upending your life, coping with it might simply entail changing the way you function in the world to compensate. Maybe you never had to keep a calendar before because everything stayed in your head, but now you've got to chart every appointment and social engagement. Small lifestyle adjustments can yield big results. One patient made a deal with her husband. If she couldn't remember someone's name at a gathering, she'd put her hand on his arm, a signal that he was to say the person's name aloud.

When Rebecca first started perimenopause, she put pads of paper everywhere—next to her computer, in the kitchen, on her bedside table—so she could scribble ideas and to-dos before they went out of her head. That's how her brain was working. She needed to write stuff down. But one thing she can say for sure is that, while her thinking was sometimes clouded, her memory not always sharp, it never impinged on her ability to do her job. She never forgot how to prescribe medication, she never forgot the names of medications, she did surgery, and she counseled patients. If anything, it made her a more sympathetic physician because she could grasp what her patients were going through.

Most likely, this will be the same for you. If you're a cashier, you can still ring people up; if you're a software engineer, you can still engineer; if you're a teacher, you can still teach. And when your brain doesn't seem to be firing on all cylinders, don't take it too seriously (remember, it's not dementia!). By the time Amy was giving that talk to her department on brain fog and her mind went blank, she was at a point where she could see the humor in it. Because sooner or later, it happens to everyone—and your perimenopausal peers will definitely get the joke.

Skin and Hair Woes

Women Take It on the Chin

My drain is so clogged right now from hair loss,
I told my husband we should buy stock in Drano.

—FORTY-EIGHT-YEAR-OLD PERIMENOPAUSAL WOMAN

Perimenopause isn't pretty, sometimes in the most literal of ways. As your hormones shift, your skin and hair will change as well. The range of aesthetic indignities that can accompany this midlife stage includes pimples popping up at the same time as lines and maybe wrinkles; dry, sandpapery skin; thinner and sometimes disappearing locks; a receding hairline; weaker nails; and sudden sprouts of chin hair. Some of these changes, like drier skin and changes to hair patterns, are part of aging, but hormonal shifts accelerate their arrival. Other changes—particularly acne—are also hormonal in nature, though not necessarily related to age. Because many of these symptoms are mostly cosmetic, they can be treated as you'd treat similar issues at almost any time of life. But the hormonal component also opens the door to other solutions.

What Happens and Why

More Than Just a Bad Hair Day

"I forget, do you part your hair on the side or in the middle?" Holly had been going to the same hairstylist for years, but the woman never remembered how she wore her wavy shoulder-length hair. But this time it was a good thing she asked: "In the middle," said Holly. In fact, Holly had always worn her hair parted on the side but now, at forty-nine, and aware that the side part was revealing a receding hairline at her upper left temple, she'd switched her part to cover it. *Oh my god*, she thought, *do I have male-pattern baldness?*

Holly's problem wasn't male-pattern baldness—it was female-pattern baldness. You don't hear that term much, but it refers to a relatively common condition that often occurs toward the end of perimenopause. While male-pattern baldness leaves the front and top of the head bare, female-pattern baldness causes the hair to recede on the sides, enhancing the widow's peak in the middle of the head. It's usually barely detectable, but you might notice it when you're combing out your hair.

Hair loss is not the only change you may be noticing. This is a time when hair texture can become coarser and a sort of "global" thinning of your tresses occurs. Amy is in the middle of this right now. Her ponytail feels as though it's half the size it once was. "Look! Can you see how thin my ponytail has become?" she said, shaking it in front of her husband. "You're insane," he replied. We're giving him a pass on this one, because hair loss often feels like a much bigger deal to you than it might to others. You might start to see more hair in your comb and in the shower drain than before, but unless you're losing it at a significant rate, it's not likely anyone else is going to spot the loss. Still, it can cause angst, especially if your hair is already feeling a little different.

As many of us know, hair changes as you get older, but the menopause transition has an impact beyond aging. The exact mechanism isn't clear. Hair follicles, the tiny organs from which hairs sprout, have sex hormone receptors that influence hair growth. In pregnancy, the increase in estrogen helps hair stay in the growing phase longer so it feels thicker. It's luxurious and full. In late-stage perimenopause, the opposite occurs. As estrogen drops, a hair follicle's growing phase shortens accordingly. There are also structural changes in the follicle that occur at this time; together the effect is to make hair fall out more quickly and feel thinner when it grows back. Estrogen also affects the amount of sebum produced by the sebaceous glands in the skin and scalp. Sebum is a waxlike substance that keeps the hair and skin lubricated; when it declines, hair becomes more brittle and breaks more easily. While these are normal signs of perimenopause, changes in hair can also be signs of low iron, and low iron itself can crop up during perimenopause if you're having heavy periods (see page 53). Changes in the hair-growth cycle and structure of the follicles affect hair on other parts of your body as well, though this can be more difficult to notice.

If you're experiencing a great deal of hair loss—you start seeing bald spots or severe receding, for instance—you may be looking at something other than a perimenopause-precipitated fallout. There is, for instance, an autoimmune condition called alopecia areata, which causes bald patches around the scalp, and another called frontal fibrosing alopecia (FFA), which makes the hair recede on the sides and the front of the head. These occur when the immune system attacks the hair follicles. Both can be accompanied by hair loss on other parts of the body, too, including the eyebrows and eyelashes. These are conditions that can affect anyone at any age, but they are often uncovered during the menopausal transition. If you recognize that your hair is disappearing appreciably, we recommend going to see a dermatologist as soon as you can, especially because FFA in particular can cause scarring so that the hair never grows back.

Another thing to be aware of is telogen effluvium, rapid hair loss caused by stress or other big life events. Telogen is the resting phase of the hair cycle and the stage where hair is shed. Most hair is in the anagen (growth) phase, but stress, medication, or physical changes can recruit a significant number of hair follicles into the telogen phase. ("Effluvium" means outflow—your hair, in other words, is outflowed off your head.) Postpartum hair loss is an example of telogen effluvium, when all that thick, luxurious hair that grew during pregnancy falls out at the same time. If you're experiencing substantial hair loss, it's good to get checked out, but we also recommend thinking about what's been happening in your life over the past several months and whether stress may be a factor.

Hair in Unexpected Places

During perimenopause, some of your body hair will start to disappear due to changes in the structure of follicles related to a drop in estrogen, but elsewhere on your body you may start to find new hairs or thicker hair than you're used to. Finding that first chin hair can be a shock, but this, too, is normal. We know of a woman who, when she reached her forties, carried a pair of tweezers with her everywhere. Even when she was idling at a stop light, she'd check the rearview mirror for chin hairs and tweeze as necessary.

These new hairs are a particular type of longer, thicker hairs, called terminal hairs, and some women also find them on their chest and abdomen during the menopausal transition. They grow in a male pattern, which is why they appear in places where men typically have hair but women don't. Everybody gets them; you just can't always see them because they're light in color, although some people get both long dark ones and long light ones. You might also find that some of your body hair gets darker during perimenopause—vellum, a type of hair that resembles peach fuzz, can become darker during this stage. How visible it becomes may depend on your hair color and ethnicity.

As with the hair on your head, the appearance of these new hairs is a result of changes in estrogen. When estrogen ebbs, testosterone, while not increasing, becomes more available. That's because when estrogen decreases so does sex hormone–binding globulin (SHGB), a big molecule that transports testosterone, holding it inactive until needed. Less SHGB means there's less opportunity to bind testosterone, so the male hormone has freer rein in the body. That's why you'll find these hairs in the same places men get them. Women with polycystic ovary syndrome (PCOS), who have higher levels of circulating androgens to begin with, are typically already fighting this pattern of hair growth. Now in perimenopause, it can get worse.

Skin and Nails

In perimenopause, the change in testosterone availability can also result in adult acne. If you were acne-prone in your youth, you may be more likely to have a recurrence now. But it can also be brand new. Welcome to your second puberty! Acne is caused by an overproduction of sebum in the hair follicles on the face. Both estrogen and testosterone contribute to oil production, but in different ways. The increase in available testosterone during this time can increase sebum secretion in specific acne-prone areas. That excess sebum combines with dead skin cells that are normally whisked out of the hair follicles through your pores and creates a bottleneck. Trapped inside, the combined sebum and dead cells allow bacteria to grow, which leads to the immune response that creates acne.

The reduction in estrogen during perimenopause actually reduces sebum production in other places, which hinders the skin's ability to hold moisture in. The resulting dryness can make you feel like you've aged overnight. But estrogen has a ton of other effects in the skin, and a decrease in estrogen can create a host of problems. The body has estrogen receptors everywhere, including every inch of skin. In the skin, estrogen helps determine thickness and "scaffolding"— provided by generous amounts of collagen, a protein that gives the skin structure. It's this architecture that makes the skin look plump and tight. Without robust scaffolding, wrinkles and lines appear.

During perimenopause, a critical element of the skin called elastin, which as its name suggests creates that bounce-back factor, also begins to wane. If you've ever noticed that the lines created by the top band of your socks leave a longer-lasting impression than they used to, you're seeing the decline of elastin.

Perimenopause is also a time when you have less blood vessel formation in your skin, which means that there are fewer "railroad tracks" to send oxygen and nutrients to where they need to go to keep your complexion looking healthy and bright. You may also see a reduction in the subcutaneous fat in your face and other parts of your body (though, sadly, not your abdomen). This fat loss causes skin to get saggy, and you can even begin to look somewhat gaunt. While this is more of an end-of-perimenopause occurrence, you may begin to see a little drooping all over.

Everyone will experience some of these changes as they age, but there's about a five-year window around perimenopause and into early menopause when it can feel like everything is changing all at once. As usual, though, there can be variations among individuals. Genetic and ethnic differences dictate either less or more visible impact from shifting hormone levels as well as the speed of skin aging overall. Lifestyle choices can make a big difference as well. Skin's appearance is also significantly shaped by long-term sun exposure and whether or not you smoked. Both do damage to the skin cells in ways that accelerate aging. Stress can affect skin, too. While we can't predict how your individual skin may change, we can say for certain that it will.

Many women also notice a change in their nails during this time. Nails are made of keratin, a protein also found in skin and hair, and during the menopausal transition, keratin is not deposited as effectively as before. As a result, you may notice that your nails—both fingernails and toenails—become thinner and lined. They may break easily, peel, or split. Like the changes to skin and hair, this is, unfortunately, a normal part of the perimenopausal process.

What You Can Do About It

While aesthetic changes may be upsetting, the good news is that there are a lot of different treatments available for each complaint, many of which you may already be familiar with.

Hair Solutions

Holly, who had developed female-pattern baldness, was essentially able to solve her problem by simply changing her part. Her hair receded no further, and she was able to hide the loss with a middle part, even though the hair at her temple unfortunately didn't grow back. That was all she needed, but when your hair loss requires more, you have a few options. The least invasive is biotin. Biotin is a B vitamin (B_7) sold as a supplement, and there are some small but not badly designed studies that show that taking somewhere between 30 and 3,000 micrograms of biotin a day can slow hair loss. If you take it in reasonable amounts, it's safe and may be effective.

You may also see biotin added to shampoos and other hair products, but biotin is not absorbed through the scalp, and there's no evidence that we know of that these products slow hair loss or induce hair growth. (If anything, you want to shampoo less often, since it strips oils from the hair.) There are also some supplements marketed as specifically designed to improve hair growth, but if you look at the label, most of them have biotin as the main ingredient. And they can be expensive. For instance, a month's supply of Nutrafol, one of the most popular hair-growth supplements (which contains biotin but also some herbal ingredients), costs about $79. But you'll only pay about $20 for a seven-month supply of biotin gummies from Costco. We prefer the gummies.

Growing hair back will require a medication like minoxidil. Minoxidil, sold under the brand name Rogaine, is a drug that spurs hair growth. It won't change a receding hairline, but it will make the areas where you still have hair fuller. It was originally developed to treat high blood pressure when the researchers noticed a side effect: hypertrichosis, or, as we know it, excessive hair growth. The mechanism behind the medication is not fully understood, but it's thought to work by increasing blood flow to the scalp and by causing the dormant hair follicles to transition into growing hair follicles. There are topical versions and oral versions of minoxidil; the topical must be applied twice a day, which is why many people prefer the oral. Pop one pill and you're done. All versions grow hair equally, but they have to be used indefinitely—once you stop using minoxidil, the hair will fall out again.

Some dermatologists also prescribe minoxidil with another drug, called spironolactone (brand name Aldactone), also originally a high blood pressure drug, which drives hair growth by acting as an anti-androgen, blocking the testosterone that contributes to receding hair. Some of our patients have heard that testosterone can stop female-pattern baldness, but this isn't true—extra testosterone will just cause more hair loss, as we see in male-pattern baldness. When it comes to hairs elsewhere on the body, like chin hairs, we recommend a good pair of tweezers and vigilant plucking, or, if you're up for it, electrolysis or laser hair removal. Spironolactone may also help here because of its ability to reduce hair follicle exposure to testosterone. Somewhat paradoxically, it can help prevent hair loss on your head while preventing hair growth on your chin.

Although we wouldn't prescribe menopausal hormone therapy for hair loss specifically, we've had patients on MHT who've anecdotally felt it helped. Despite the enthusiasm, it's unclear whether MHT has a significant effect on hair loss in women. If it does have an effect, it's certainly not a quick fix. If you're having hot flashes or mood issues because of perimenopause, we expect to see improvements from MHT in a matter of weeks. The fix for hair loss (and it stops the loss, rather than making it grow back) is more of a slow burn. It may take six to twelve months before you see improvement, if you see improvement at all.

Birth control pills don't seem to have much of an effect on hair loss, but may have a small impact on the chin hair problem. Certain types of contraception contain drospirenone (a type of progestin that works at the progesterone receptor), which, like spironolactone, has anti-androgenic properties and so may prevent some of that testosterone-driven, male-like hair sprouting. More specifically, drospirenone works by elevating SHGB, which ties up testosterone so there's less of it available in the body.

Skin Fixes

While hormones may or may not stem hair loss, we have better data to suggest that estrogen can slow skin aging. Some research, for instance, shows that estrogen taken as a pill (allowing it to go throughout the body) can improve the thickness of the skin within six months. A 2023 review of skin rejuvenation in women using MHT also found that hormonal therapy improved both collagen content and elasticity in the skin. We should note that other research doesn't indicate that there are any skin benefits to MHT, but anecdotally, many of our patients report an improvement in skin and nails when taking it. Birth control pills aren't as likely to stop the wrinkling and dryness as hormone therapy, but they do have an impact on acne. Just as the drospirenone in contraception helps stop chin hair growth by lowering testosterone exposure, so, too, does it block the androgen-induced acne that can crop up in perimenopause.

If hormones are so effective at helping the skin, you may wonder whether a hormonal face cream could be beneficial. We've seen face creams that contain estrogen advertised online, but it's not clear that they help—and they may even cause harm. One study looked at three sample groups—one using a face cream with estradiol, one with estriol, and one with no estrogen. (Estradiol, as you may recall, is a form of estrogen made primarily in the ovaries; estriol is a form made mostly by the placenta when you're pregnant.) According to the dermatologist assessing the skin on the study subjects' faces, both estrogen groups had "statistically significant" improvement in overall facial aging, slightly better than those given only lotion. But when they asked the women what they thought, equal numbers of women in each group thought they looked better after applying a moisturizer for twelve weeks, even those who didn't have any estrogen in the formulation they were using.

So there may be a slight benefit to using estrogen-containing face cream, but is it safe? Skin absorbs estrogen easily—this is why we try to be careful when prescribing estrogen creams for vaginal dryness—so we wanted to know whether any of the women in the study showed higher levels of estrogen from using the face cream. The study found that the estriol-containing cream did not raise blood estrogen levels, but there was a slight bump in estradiol. It wasn't enough to set off alarm bells; however, the study was only twelve weeks long, and estrogen has the potential to build up over time. If you're putting it on your face, you're not going to just do it for three months and stop; you're going to keep going. How will estrogen levels change over time? We don't know the answer to that question, and that gives us pause. Also, it is important to note the study was too small for us to be sure of this result, so many more women would have to be studied for us to know this is safe.

When we prescribe localized, topical estrogen—for vaginal dryness, not for the face—we also go about it in a safe manner and with confidence that it has been well studied. The research tells us that topical estrogen is not absorbed significantly from the vagina, possibly because the vagina is toward the end of your blood supply. Although you absorb estrogen through the vaginal walls, the vagina is sort of like a river delta. Not much is actually going to flow back up into your body, whereas your face is much more mid-river, with estrogen flowing down. The face also has a larger surface area than the vagina—and thus more of an absorption zone—plus it's difficult to control the dosage when you're slathering on a cream. Vaginal estrogen, on the other hand, is dosed very specifically, at very low levels. (This refers specifically to estrogen suppositories, which is what we prescribe, rather than estrogen creams, though they are also available. In fact, we have had patients report that they use their vaginal estrogen cream on their face. Don't do this!)

The bottom line is that, in our opinion, topical estrogen moisturizers are not ready for prime time. We don't know enough yet about their long-term effects to recommend them. The other issue that keeps us from endorsing estrogen face creams is that the study didn't show that they had any benefit over just regular lotion. Women on both sides of the study shared that they felt their skin looked better, and it's true that using a good lotion can go a long way to mitigate some of the negative effects perimenopause can have on your skin. A moisturizer with hyaluronic acid, which binds water to skin cells, can help combat the dryness you may now be experiencing. There are a ton of options—choose the one that works best for your skin and budget. Moisturizing your nail beds can even help with some of perimenopause's effects on your nails, though you may need to add in a nail strengthener serum to really see a difference. Regardless, adding moisture to your skin and body during this time is one of the simplest ways to combat the sudden changes you may be seeing.

Like moisturizer, sunscreen is an easy addition to your perimenopausal toolkit. It's possible that some of the changes you're noticing in your skin are due not to perimenopause but to long-term sun exposure. "I like to differentiate between photoaging and chronological aging," says Sonja M. Krejci, MD, a dermatologist at the Seattle Clinical Research Center. "Many of the changes that are attributed to accumulating birthdays are primarily the result of photodamage. You can see it when you look at the difference between the skin on your chest and the skin on your buttocks." The changes Dr. Krejci is talking about include freckling, brown spots, red or purple lines, fine wrinkling, and sallowness. "So the best product to make skin appear more youthful is a good broad-spectrum sunscreen together with hats, clothing, and seeking shade." It doesn't matter which sunscreen you use as long as it feels comfortable on your skin, you use it every day, and it's got a high-enough sun protection factor (SPF—go for 30 or higher) to help you defend against UV damage.

Even if you don't mind the aesthetic effects of photodamage, we strongly recommend using sunscreen because of the risk of skin cancer. By the time you reach midlife, you may have accumulated years of sun damage (especially if you grew up in a place where slathering yourself with oil and "laying out" was pretty normal behavior). For that reason, and especially if skin cancer runs in your family, it's a good idea to check to make sure any moles you have are not cancerous. (See "The ABCDE's of Melanoma.") If you're prone to moles, you should be having a dermatologist check you yearly.

THE ABCDE'S OF MELANOMA

Survey the moles on your body (or better yet have someone else do it for you). If you see any of these signs, see a dermatologist.

A is for Asymmetry. Most moles are uniformly round; oddly shaped ones need to be assessed.

B is for Border. Melanoma borders tend to be uneven and not smooth like normal moles.

C is for Color. Multiple colors are a warning sign. Benign moles are usually a single shade of brown.

D is for Diameter or Dark. If a mole is the size of a pencil eraser (about 6 mm, or ¼ inch in diameter) or larger and very dark, no matter what size it is, get it checked out.

E is for Evolving. Any change in size, shape, color, or elevation of a spot on your skin, or any new symptom, such as bleeding, itching, or crusting, may be a warning sign of melanoma.

Another consequence of perimenopausal skin changes is an increase in sensitivity. As you're considering your skincare routine at this age, keep in mind that your skin may be more delicate than it was in the past. When it comes to facial cleansers, avoid those that contain soap, which is not only harsh but washes away protective oils. Look for a cleanser that's oil-based, or consider just washing your face with water. It may feel weird if you're used to a very particular cleansing routine, but sometimes it's all you need. If you do require something with a little more gravitas—say you need to take off makeup—consider cold cream or something similar. Also, as you shop for skincare, keep in mind that things like added fragrance, essential oils, and other unnecessary ingredients are more likely to irritate your skin than help it. Simple is going to be kindest to your midlife skin.

What about anti-aging ingredients? Alpha hydroxy acids such as glycolic acid (and others: lactic, malic, citric, mandelic, and tartaric acids) can be beneficial as exfoliants. They remove dead, complexion-dulling skin cells and can improve skin texture and color and help with acne breakouts. There's also good evidence to suggest that retinoids, such as tretinoin and to a lesser extent its lower-strength cousin retinol, help reduce fine lines and wrinkles, lighten dark spots, and improve the color and texture of the skin. Retinoids are also often prescribed for acne, so something to think about if you're having perimenopausal-induced flare-ups.

The downside of these products is that they can be very irritating. Retinoids and retinol can cause redness, flakiness, and burning, especially if your skin has become more sensitive than before. Retinoids still require a prescription in the United States (retinols are available in over-the-counter formulations) and are available in multiple potencies and vehicles depending on individual needs. A dermatologist can provide guidance on proper use and progression in strength to avoid irritation and a condition called retinoid dermatitis. Even if you're only using a retinol product, take it slow. See how your skin responds—the side effects may eventually subside—and go from there.

Another product you may have heard used for anti-aging is vitamin C. "Use of vitamin C in the morning paired with a retinoid at night is also a great combination for treating photoaging and maintaining healthy skin," says Dr. Krejci. "Vitamin C functions as an antioxidant and neutralizes free radicals that are damaging to the skin." Unfortunately, it can be difficult to find a product with potent vitamin C since it's very unstable and difficult to package while maintaining potency. "It can be overwhelming trying to select high-quality products with proven effective and potent ingredients," says Dr. Krejci. "One thing to know, though, is that you do not always get a better product by paying a lot more money because a good portion of the cost is from marketing and packaging and not necessarily the individual ingredients." Look to your dermatologist or an aesthetician (especially ones who work together with a dermatologist) for good recommendations on products. And when in doubt, just make sure you have a moisturizer and sunscreen that you like and will use. Those are the most important things.

11

Hot Flashes and Night Sweats

Swelter Skelter

I once got a hot flash in response to hearing food sizzling
in the microwave. Just the thought of heat!

—FIFTY-FIVE-YEAR-OLD POSTMENOPAUSAL WOMAN

First, it was the silk scarf around her neck that came off. Next Amira slowly unbelted and removed her jacket. She tossed the navy blazer with the cinched waist onto a chair. Then, the situation cried out for more, so she began unbuttoning her blouse, baring the tank top underneath. As you might have guessed—this is a chapter on hot flashes, after all—the undressing wasn't meant to be a sexy striptease. Amira, president of a biotech company, was in the middle of giving a presentation to the all-male board as her assistant looked on in what-are-you-doing disbelief. After the meeting, Amira seriously thought about quitting her job. "I used to really command the boardroom," she says. "I didn't feel like I could do that anymore."

Hot flashes are one of the most notorious symptoms of the menopausal transition. They can cause distress in every area of life—disruptive to sleep, distracting to the brain, and diminishing to the ego. It can be embarrassing to have rivulets of sweat running down your face when everyone else around you is as cool as a 7-Eleven Slurpee, but these stressful episodes are incredibly common, though they may vary in severity and frequency depending on the individual. It's estimated that 75 to 80 percent of women in the United States experience hot flashes during this time, while globally hot flashes are reported in about 57 percent of women. And the incidence and severity seem to differ among nations. According to one study, women in Turkey are the most likely to suffer hot flashes, with rates as elevated as 97 percent, the highest incidence in the world. In Australia, it's not so much the number of vasomotor symptoms—the technical term for hot flashes, which are also sometimes referred to as hot flushes—as the intensity: Australians seem to get the most ferocious flashes and sweats.

The length of time a woman experiences hot flashes can also vary—and can depend on her race, weight, and a range of other factors. The average span of hot flashes among women in the United States is 7.4 years, but research shows that Black women suffer hot flashes longer—a median of 10 years. Hispanic and Black women also have a higher incidence of suffering from hot flashes than white women. Of the First Nations women who were studied by a group of researchers at Northern Ontario School of Medicine (NOSM) in Sioux Lookout, Ontario, only half the women had vasomotor symptoms.

Chinese American and Japanese American women also tend to be less likely to suffer hot flashes, which may have something to do with body fat. Body fat keeps heat in, an advantage if you're out in the cold, but a disadvantage during the menopausal transition. In general, Asian people tend to be on the leaner side of the body fat spectrum, which may account for why they report less struggle with hot flashes. Obese women, on the other hand, have a higher likelihood of severe hot flashes. No matter your body type, though, the experience of having hot flashes is pretty universally frustrating.

That said, hot flashes don't tend to be the biggest complaint for perimenopausal women. In part, this is because they tend to arrive later in perimenopause, as you get closer to menopause. Early on, you may not even realize you're having hot flashes, because they usually begin at night. If you're having trouble sleeping due to night sweats or temperature issues, you're probably starting to have hot flashes—night sweats are hot flashes that happen when you're asleep. Because they occur when you're unconscious, they tend to feel different. Some women just feel overly warm and throw off the covers. Some get all the way through a hot flash without feeling the heat, then wake up drenched and cold asking themselves, *What just happened?* When a hot flash comes on during the day, you can adjust, strip off layers like Amira did, put yourself in front of a fan, or gulp down a glass of ice water. In sleep, you have no real options other than to toss off blankets or sweat.

One patient, Theresa, had a particularly dramatic experience with night sweats. When Theresa was forty-six, she started to wake up a little damp. After a year or so of this, dampness turned to soggy, and she had to keep a spare pair of pajamas next to her bed to change into. She asked the nurse practitioner she was seeing if it could be perimenopause. "She said no, it was 'just stress,'" remembers Theresa. Then one night she noticed that her pajama bottoms were moister than her shirt. She had had incontinence in the past but had pelvic floor physical therapy and the problem went away. Now she thought immediately, *Uh-oh, the incontinence has come back.*

Theresa returned to the medical practice and this time saw a different nurse practitioner, who prescribed medication for incontinence. But it didn't stop the nighttime wetness, and she was now having to sleep on top of towels and change her pajamas at least once a night. Because the medication obviously wasn't working, she stopped taking it. And things just got worse to the point where she began wearing an adult diaper at night—but even that didn't work! "I would wake up with the Depends completely dry, but the bed was still soaked! I thought, do

I need a different brand? Are they the wrong size? Why weren't they working?" says Theresa. What was stranger was that none of the soaking wet pajamas or towels smelled like urine.

Four years into this nightmare, Theresa took herself to a urologist at a local university hospital who specialized in women's incontinence. While in the waiting room, passing the time looking at her laptop, she decided to search Google for advice on how to explain what was happening to her to the doctor. She searched "soaked from neck to knees." Guess what came up? Perimenopause.

Theresa proceeded with the urologist appointment. Her bladder was injected with, as the nurse put it, "more liquid than most women your age can hold," and she was told to cough and push. Nothing came out. She showed the search results on her laptop to the doctor. "Could this be perimenopause?" "Yes!" affirmed the doctor. In her earlier appointments with the nurse practitioners, Theresa was told she couldn't possibly be in perimenopause because, according to her blood tests, her estrogen level was "normal." (This is exactly why we advise against blood tests for perimenopause—see page 12.) "I now know that the lower part of my anatomy sweats a lot more than the upper part during hot flashes," says Theresa. "It was awful driving around in a car with leather seats in the summer. It felt like sitting in a swimming pool."

Admittedly, this is an unusual story, so if you haven't started having night sweats or hot flashes in the daytime yet, don't panic. In the early years of perimenopause, you may even have hot flashes that come and go. Amy had a patient who booked an appointment because she was having hot flashes, only to have them disappear by the time her appointment arrived. "I didn't have my period for a few months, and I started having hot flashes," she said. "But then my periods resumed, and they went away." Because of fluctuating estrogen levels, this is a not-uncommon part of the perimenopausal roller-coaster ride. But as menopause nears and estrogen stays low instead of ping-ponging up and down, regular hot flashes can set in.

What's Happening and Why

Until about fifteen years ago, science had turned up no explanation for why women suffer from hot flashes. And we still don't know why some women get them and some women don't and why, beyond a body fat connection, they vary in severity. For a long time, scientists believed the symptoms were related to estrogen's effect on the vascular system, which makes sense because when the body becomes hot, blood rushes to your face, limbs, and other parts of your body, dilating the blood vessels to help cool you off. Now, however, we know that hot flashes are all about brain wiring, and physical responses like vasodilation and perspiration are responses to the "heat" the body thinks it's experiencing, even if there are no external factors.

Temperature regulation in the human body is controlled by the hypothalamus, a structure in the brain that holds sway not only over temperature but blood pressure, mood, hunger, sex drive, sleep, and more. The hypothalamus receives messages from neurons across the brain and body, and tells other neurons how to respond. We now believe that the root cause of hot flashes as you approach menopause is changes in those messages.

GnRH neurons are one of many kinds of neurons in the hypothalamus. GnRH, as you might remember from chapter 2, is a messenger that pulses in varying ways to communicate different directives. One of its important functions is to order the release of follicle-stimulating hormone (FSH) to prompt the ovaries to prepare a viable egg for fertilization. When a viable egg is produced, the egg sends estrogen back to the brain and GnRH quiets down. But when you are well into perimenopause and the ovaries are having trouble developing that viable egg, there's no estrogen response, which causes GnRH to pulse faster and faster, knocking harder and harder because no one is coming to the door.

In the middle of all this is a type of neuron called KNDy (kisspeptin, neurokinin B, and dynorphin A). In response to the pulsing of GnRH, these neurons start firing and firing and firing, too, affecting a third type of neuron called warm-sensitive neurons. The warm-sensitive neurons are responsible for telling the hypothalamus what the normal temperature range for the body is. But with all these excitable neurons firing its way, it narrows that range, making the hypothalamus unusually sensitive to temperature. Anytime the body goes out of that now-minuscule range, it becomes convinced it's too hot and triggers vasodilation and sweating, creating what you know as a hot flash.

Unlike when you go outside on a hot day and get all red-faced and sweaty, there's no external stimulus causing the warm-sensitive neurons to trigger your cooling-off measures. It's like that old urban legend where the babysitter gets a threatening phone call only to find out *the call is coming from inside the house!* The stimulus for a hot flash is coming from inside your brain, asking your body to let out as much heat as possible. And the body can release a shocking amount of heat—one patient reported that her husband could feel the heat from her night sweats on the other side of the bed.

The good news is that these episodes are likely temporary. GnRH neurons eventually give up and stop their manic pulsing, and everything quiets down. As you get further away from your final menstrual period, your hot flashes will likely taper off. Studies show that about 80 percent of women report that their hot flashes eventually went away, although it doesn't happen immediately; in fact it could take up to seven to ten years before they taper to a final stop (and some women, we're sorry to reveal, never lose them altogether). Unfortunately, the earlier you start hot flashing, the more likely they are to hang on longer. The hot flashes are also more likely to be of greater intensity and more frequent.

You could argue that there's some evolutionary reasoning behind menopause (see page 18), but there doesn't seem to be any Darwinian rationale behind hot flashes (as far as we know). It's likely that they're a mistake. Hot flashes don't help perpetuate the species in any way, and they're actually associated with increased risk: Women who have hot flashes longer and also flash intensely are more likely to have cardiovascular disease later in life. One of the SWAN studies found that women with more severe hot flashes had a 50 to 77 percent increased risk of cardiovascular events such as heart attacks, strokes, and heart failure. This sounds scary but we don't know that it's a case of cause and effect. We only know that there's an association. Nonetheless, if your hot flashes have started early and are fierce, you and your physician need to keep an eye on your heart health as you grow older.

PERSISTENT PERSPIRATION: HOT FLASHES THAT DON'T GO AWAY

A rare subset of women, known as super flashers or persistent flashers, will experience hot flashes that don't go away, to the extent that they can make life unmanageable. Amanda was one of these super flashers. She began having hot flashes in perimenopause when she was in her late forties, and began menopausal hormone therapy to treat them in her fifties. MHT really helped, and for many years she was fine. But after she'd been on estrogen for about ten years, her primary care doctor recommended that she come off it due to age-related risks of MHT (see page 189 for more on this). He assumed her hot flashes would have ebbed by then. They hadn't. Instead, they came back with a vengeance. Amanda began having four to five hot flashes an hour and they were drenching. At night, she had to change her sheets four times before morning. Things were so bad that she got an accommodation from her job to work from home, where she could keep her thermostat at a cool 60 degrees. But Amanda basically became agoraphobic. She was afraid to go out because she feared she'd start flashing in front of people.

Amanda went back to her doctor and asked to resume MHT, but the doctor refused to prescribe it to her because she was now sixty-three. "It's just a quality of life thing," he said, as if quality of life was not anything to be concerned about. Amanda suffered for two more years, before coming in to see Rebecca. "I don't want to live," she said. "I'll kill myself if this doesn't stop." This is an instance when a physician and a patient together have to weigh the risks against the benefits. Amanda was not at high risk for breast cancer or heart disease, and her distress was not to be taken lightly. The solution was pretty clear. Rebecca prescribed estrogen, and Amanda got her life back. She returned to working in the office, she could sleep again, and she was no longer afraid to go out.

Hot flashes have become the world's favorite menopause joke, and we can laugh about them—but when you're experiencing them, they're not very funny. It really is okay to ask for help to make them go away, especially if you're among the women whose flashes are unrelenting.

What You Can Do About It

If you're already experiencing night sweats and/or hot flashes, you're probably aware of some of the obvious strategies: dress in layers, carry a fan, keep the thermostat low, try a device that cools your bed like the Chilipad we talked about in chapter 4. There's also another product, called BedJet, which blows cool air on one side of the bed and can similarly help regulate sleeping temperature. It may help, too, if you sleep on a regular mattress versus a memory foam mattress—the latter type tends to trap body heat. You can also buy "cooling pajamas for hot sleepers" or try different sheets, but at a certain point you may want a stronger solution.

Your next instinct may be to try a nonhormonal therapy like black cohosh, which is an herbal supplement, or soy isoflavones, a supplement derived from soybeans. We always tell our patients that they're welcome to try any of the alternative treatments; maybe they'll help, but it's a big maybe. The Menopause Society, a professional group to which we both belong, has vetted research on black cohosh, as well as wild yam, dong quai, evening primrose, maca, ginseng, chasteberry, milk thistle, omega-3 fatty acids, and vitamin E, and found that they mostly work no better than a placebo. That said, placebos do work 20 to 30 percent of the time, so any of these may provide some relief for a while.

The Menopause Society does not recommend soy, but we think it might be worth a try because there's some data to suggest limited efficacy. Isoflavones can be converted to an active form of estrogen that binds to the estrogen receptors in the body. A review of supplementation with equol (a converted form of isoflavones) has found some benefit in reduction of hot flashes. However, not everyone can metabolize soy into the active, receptor-binding form. People in Asia, for instance, have a much higher conversion rate than people in Europe and North America (maybe another reason they seem less susceptible to hot flashes). Most herbal supplements sold in grocery stores are not going to hurt you, but there are a few things we want to note and a few we want you to avoid if you decide to take them—we'll discuss supplements and offer some general advice on purchasing and using them in chapter 14.

Among the other alternative treatments we have had patients try is acupuncture. The research on acupuncture for hot flashes is mixed, with some small studies showing an effect and other, larger studies showing no effect. It may depend on who's doing the acupuncture and how skilled they are (no matter who you see, make sure that they sterilize the needles!). There's also a variation on acupuncture called electroacupuncture, which involves small electrodes attached to the needles. In one small study, that showed some promise in treating hot flashes. It's not a miracle cure, but at the very least, lying on a table while waiting for the acupuncture to work can be very meditative. And meditation may help with other symptoms you're experiencing. But we'd be neglectful if we didn't add that meditation, as well as yoga and other forms of exercise, doesn't show appreciable benefits where hot flashes are concerned. Nonetheless, these are all low-risk modalities worth a try and, as noted, may help you with other perimenopausal symptoms like anxiety and sleep disturbances.

There are a few other nonpharmaceutical treatments that have shown effectiveness for hot flashes. In a review of studies presented at a meeting of the Menopause Society in 2024, researchers from Baylor University determined that hypnotherapy (also called clinical hypnosis) reduced hot flash frequency by 60 percent. And hypnosis had a real impact on the women's day-to-day, improving sleep, mood, and other aspects of their lives. The researchers also found that the round of studies, published between 1996 and 2022, showed that cognitive behavioral therapy, while only reducing frequency minimally, reduced the stress associated with hot flashes.

The most proven remedy for hot flashes is hormone therapy. In fact, it's been approved by the FDA for hot flash treatment since 1942. When your brain is replenished with estrogen via hormone therapy, the neurons that trigger vasomotor symptoms quiet down, mitigating hot flash severity or stopping them entirely. This is something you might consider if hot flashes are interfering with your work, your ability to care for your family and others, your social relationships, your stress levels, or just your overall well-being. There's no litmus test for choosing MHT to treat hot flashes—if they're bothering you, and there are low risks to taking MHT, it may be the perfect solution. Your doctor will be able to help you decide if MHT is right for your situation.

When we prescribe hormone therapy for hot flashes, we like to set expectations. Research shows that estrogen therapy can reduce the severity and frequency of hot flashes by 65 to 90 percent whether or not it's taken with progesterone (a precautionary add-in for women who have a uterus, meant to avoid the buildup of the uterus lining from extra estrogen). It's not likely that taking estrogen will reduce hot flashes to zero, especially if you're having several hot flashes an hour and stripping your bedsheets in the middle of the night. Many women find that MHT can reduce hot flashes to the point where you can get things done; you can manage without feeling overtaxed, miserable, and embarrassed. "I haven't had night sweats or 'incontinence' since being on MHT," says Theresa. And it's not just "quality of life": When hot flashes interfere with your sleep and raise your stress level, they're a detriment to your health as well. (See chapter 14 for more on MHT.)

Although hormonal treatments are a frequent choice for treating hot flashes, some women are not candidates for MHT, and some just prefer not to take hormones. For these women, we can look to nonhormonal medications that have been proven to help. In 2023, the FDA approved Veozah (fezolinetant), a drug specifically developed to treat hot flashes. Veozah blocks the excitable KNDy neurons' neurokinin B from knocking the warm-sensitive neurons into high gear, which helps the brain reestablish regular temperature control. Rather than covering up the symptoms, as some nonhormonal medications can do, Veozah gets to the root of the problem. The medication has few side effects (some people experience headaches), but it works pretty well across studies, reducing hot flashes by about 70 percent. It also works pretty quickly, so you'll know within the first few weeks if it's the right choice for you.

As we were writing this book, another KNDy-blocking drug, called elinzanetant, was being vetted for FDA approval. So far, the results of studies done on elinzanetant show that it significantly reduced the frequency and intensity of hot flashes. It's also been found to improve sleep and may even work better than Veozah. We're hopeful that the development of these drugs is a sign that pharmaceutical companies are finally waking up to the value of developing drugs specifically for problems facing women.

Other drugs that work on the brain can help with hot flashes as well. Antidepressants have shown an effectiveness rate of 45 to 50 percent, and because they're typically prescribed at low doses when given just for hot flashes, the side effects are minimal (although if you're also having mood issues, your doctor might prescribe them at a higher dose to treat both mood and hot flashes). The ones most commonly used for their vasomotor effects are paroxetine (Paxil, Pexeva) and venlafaxine (Effexor XR). Brisdelle, a low-dose form of paroxetine, is actually FDA-approved for the treatment of hot flashes. The other antidepressants are prescribed off-label (that is, at the discretion of your doctor).

It's important to discuss the different options with a healthcare provider because there are some medications that interfere with each other. When a woman is taking tamoxifen for breast cancer, for instance, we have to be careful about what we prescribe because certain antidepressants can hinder the activation of the drug. If you're taking tamoxifen, this may be a time when your doctor will look at other medications that can help with hot flashes. As a general rule, it's essential to bring up *all* your perimenopausal symptoms when talking to your doctor about hot flashes. You might be able to treat hot flashes with one nonhormonal drug, but it won't help you solve the other seven symptoms you may have. The more birds you can hit with one stone, the better. We'll take a deeper dive into your treatment options in part 3.

Part Three

Comprehensive Treatments

Contraception.
Yep, Contraception!

Why You Might Need It Now

When I told my doctor about my symptoms, he offered me birth control pills. Birth control pills! I feel like he was blowing me off.

—FORTY-THREE-YEAR-OLD PERIMENOPAUSAL WOMAN

Although you may feel you no longer need or want to take birth control, we do ask that you remain open-minded. It might be just the ticket to address your symptoms at this time. Despite what you may have read or heard on social media, your doctor is not necessarily blowing you off by suggesting this as a therapy, but they may not be doing a great job of explaining *why* this might be a great option for you. That's where we come in—we want to help you understand the *why* so you can decide if this is the right option for you.

Birth control pills can be an effective treatment for many of the symptoms of perimenopause. But it isn't just pills that can be useful—any hormone-based form of contraception, including intrauterine devices (IUDs), can be an effective way to treat perimenopausal symptoms, some more comprehensively than others. In the early to middle years of perimenopause, when hormone levels are bobbing up and down like horses on a carousel, some contraceptives, such as combined hormonal birth control pills, can regulate those volatile hormones and have a calming effect on associated symptoms, like irregular periods, mood swings, acne, and even hot flashes.

Let's start with the obvious. Contraception provides . . . contraception. Remember, until you've gone a year without a period, you can still conceive. And many women at midlife do. When you look at pregnancy demographics, the women with the highest rate of unintended pregnancies are teenagers *and* women in their forties. In 2023, the National Center for Health Statistics published a report updating the data on pregnancy, both intended and unintended. Overall, unintended pregnancies declined from 43 to 41 percent, but the rate of unplanned pregnancies in women over forty didn't dip; in fact, it rose slightly. This isn't to say that it's easy to conceive during this time, but it is possible. For women ages forty to forty-four, the risk of pregnancy is 10 percent; for women ages forty-five to forty-nine, it's 2 to 3 percent. So if you're not trying to get pregnant, hormonal birth control can be a great way to avoid an accidental pregnancy while helping you feel better at the same time.

You may be surprised to hear us recommend birth control as treatment for perimenopause, especially if you've seen discussions of the drawbacks of different kinds of birth control, like the pill and IUDs. While we want to emphasize that the risk of pregnancy doesn't go away at this age, we recognize that for many women in perimenopause, contraception isn't a core concern. Why would we recommend birth control, with its supposed risks, before something designed to treat menopausal symptoms, like MHT?

There are two parts to this answer. First, let's talk about the alleged drawbacks of hormonal birth control. While there are some risks with hormonal treatments, which we'll discuss in detail later in this chapter, hormonal treatments in general are very safe, and much of the negative information you may have heard about them is likely exaggerated or misstated. Of course, we always take into account patients' symptoms, medical history, and need for contraception to make the right recommendation for them. But unless you are at special risk for specific negative side effects, there are few drawbacks to hormonal birth control, and a lot to be gained.

As to the second question, there are some important differences between hormonal birth control and MHT. Hormonal birth control uses either a combination of estrogen and progestogen or a form of progestogen alone to prevent ovulation and the hormonal instability that comes with it, thereby regulating the menstrual cycle (as we will explain in greater detail later in this chapter). Hormonal therapies designed for the menopausal transition use similar hormones in different dosages to specifically target perimenopause and menopause symptoms, but MHT does not have the added (and extremely important) benefit of contraception, and it does not stop ovulation or the crazy hormonal fluctuations that result from the tired ovaries trying to ovulate. If you're using MHT during perimenopause, the ovaries continue to function on top of the MHT, and you might still get symptoms such as mood instability and heavy periods because the hormonal fluctuations are still present. These fluctuations may not be as severe as they were at baseline because the MHT stops the big drops, but it doesn't stop the big peaks like combined hormonal contraception does. That's why this therapy might be better for you at this time.

Later, as you get closer to menopause and the roller-coastering hormones settle down, you may be better served by MHT. But in these earlier stages, we often recommend birth control as a way to kill two birds with one stone. Of course, some women prefer to skip comprehensive hormone-based treatments altogether and treat their symptoms individually or use a comprehensive remedy that doesn't contain hormones. We'll look at all these options in the coming chapters. We will, however, start the conversation by explaining the use of birth control in perimenopause, just as we usually do during our office visits.

How It Helps

Combined Hormonal Contraception

Most hormone-based birth control pills, patches, and rings fall into a category known as combined hormonal contraception. That is, they contain a combination of varying forms of estrogen and progestins (a type of progestogen that works at the progesterone receptor). There are some hormonal contraceptives (certain pills and IUDs) that contain only progestins, which work differently than combined forms of hormones but can also help manage symptoms. We'll get to those later down the line.

Together, estrogen and progestin prevent conception by effectively shutting down ovulation. The estrogen in combined hormonal methods causes the brain to suppress the production of follicle-stimulating hormone so that the ovaries don't receive the usual prompt to start the monthly process of developing an egg suitable for fertilization. The progestin prevents the usual surge in luteinizing hormone, the messenger that tells the body to release the egg down the fallopian tube. It also makes the uterus an unwelcome place for an embryo and thickens cervical mucus, making it difficult for sperm to get through to the uterus.

In this process of preventing ovulation, combined hormone contraception also turns off the hormonal roller coaster responsible for so many perimenopausal symptoms, most especially heavy and unpredictable periods. While taking it, you're likely to have a lighter flow and fewer days of bleeding. You can even choose the type of pills that allow you to have a period only a few times a year or not at all, reducing the bleeding to almost nothing. If you're prone to bad bouts of PMS or even premenstrual dysphoric disorder (PMDD), the severest form of PMS, combined hormonal birth control will likely help with those symptoms as well.

For some women, stopping the symptoms related to menstruation alone can be life-changing. Melissa is a woman who never had an easy menstrual cycle. PMS had always led to deeply unsettling mood swings; then when the bleeding began, she'd have terrible cramps and feel completely exhausted. From the time she hit puberty, about a week and a half of every month was misery. Then when Melissa turned fifty-one, a week and a half turned into what felt like PMS every day. "I went through a pretty hairy few months but had a doctor who put me on low-dose birth control pills," she says. "I took them for three months and it helped a lot." Once Melissa fully hit menopause, all her period-related symptoms stopped, but the birth control was a crucial tool for helping her weather the transition in between.

Combined hormonal birth control is also reliably helpful for reducing or eliminating a number of other perimenopause symptoms. In the absence of hormonal swings, mood swings often disappear. Menstrual migraines, which for many women occur in the week leading up to their period, when estradiol drops off, and which can get worse in perimenopause, may be reduced as well. A recent study also found that women in their forties taking combined hormonal birth control pills had reduced hot flashes, less depression and anxiety, and fewer headaches. The pills boosted their interest in sex, too. For three months, researchers had thirty-four women cycle through combined hormone pills for twenty-one days, with two days of placebo tablets and five days of an estrogen-only tablet. Twenty-six other women took twenty-one days' worth of the same pills, but with seven placebo tablets. All the women reaped the symptom-relief benefits noted above, and the women who received the extra estrogen fared even better. (We'll discuss the pros and cons of estrogen later.)

Progestin-Only Contraception

Progestin-only birth control—meaning it contains no estrogen—primarily prevents pregnancy by thickening the cervical mucus so sperm can't get in. This type of contraception, whether in pill or IUD form, can be very effective at reducing heavy perimenopausal menstrual bleeding. That means it can give you relief if your periods are alarmingly and uncomfortably torrential. Progestin-only birth control generally doesn't prevent ovulation (though a few types do) and on its own may not treat other perimenopausal symptoms, but can still be a helpful part of the therapy equation. We'll talk more about why you might choose a progestin-only birth control, and how they help and their pros and cons, later in this chapter.

Making Sense of the Choices

Like most medications, birth control is not a one-size-fits-all solution, and there is a wide range of available choices, which allows doctors like us to tailor contraception to our perimenopausal patients' particular symptoms, while also taking into consideration other health issues, personal preferences (some people, for instance, hate taking pills), and even what's covered by insurers. You and your doctor can decide what makes the most sense for you, and if the first prescription you try doesn't work, there are a lot of other options available to you.

Birth Control Pills

When people refer to birth control pills or "the pill," they usually mean combined hormonal contraception that contains both estrogen and progestin. (As noted, there are birth control pills that are progestin-only pills, which we'll discuss shortly.) The birth control pill, which one could argue changed life as we know it (the *Economist* once called it "one of the Seven Wonders of the Modern World"), was decades in the making. Its creation picked up speed in 1941 when it was discovered that Mexican women had long been using a particular variety of wild yam to prevent conception. The yam contained diosgenin, a type of estrogen that can be converted to a progestin, then extracted and combined with estrogen to fabricate an effective form of birth control. Years of clinical trials followed, and, finally, in 1957, the FDA approved the pill—ironically, to regulate menstruation. In 1960, the FDA weighed in again, approving the pill for contraceptive purposes. By 1967, 13 million women across the world were on the pill.

While the pill was effective, it was not without side effects. The most worrisome was an increased risk of heart attack, stroke, and deep vein thrombosis (blood clots). But then researchers found that the original pill's hormone content—10,000 micrograms of progestin and 150 micrograms of estrogen—was far higher than needed to deter pregnancy, and the risks could be reduced by lowering these dosages. Pharmaceutical companies have now spent generations turning down the dosage and tinkering with different forms of the hormones. The currently available lower-dose pills can have anywhere from 50 to 150 micrograms of progestin and 20 to 50 micrograms of estrogen (there are even pills with estrogen as low as 10 micrograms), which substantially reduces the likelihood of dangerous side effects.

While the pill still carries a very small risk of heart attack, stroke, high blood pressure, and blood clots, the benefits often far outweigh the danger. Unwanted pregnancy, for example, doesn't just pose a difficult life decision—it's a huge undertaking for the body that carries its own risks, including a major increase in the risk of blood clots and other concerns. Combined hormonal birth control pills also have beneficial health effects for women beyond pregnancy prevention and mitigating perimenopause symptoms: They have been shown to help prevent bone loss and even to enhance bone density, as well as lower the risk of endometrial and colorectal cancers. Research has also found that the risk of ovarian cancer drops as much as 50 percent for women on the pill, and that the protection lasts for years after you stop taking them.

These are additional variables your doctor will consider before prescribing a birth control pill or possibly offering you an alternative. If you have other risk factors for blood clots, like a family history or smoking, or if you've had or have a hormone-sensitive cancer like breast or ovarian, there are nonhormonal options that might be a better fit for you. Some people just don't respond well to combined hormone pills, which usually contain a type of estrogen called ethinyl estradiol that can have side effects like bloating, nausea, and breast tenderness. Research on alternative estrogens is ongoing, and some new formulations of pills are already showing promise.

Age is also a consideration when it comes to the pill being a fit for some women, with current wisdom being that patients can take the pill until age fifty-five. Even that guideline is more of a suggestion than a rule, based on the fact that most women are in menopause by fifty-five and no longer need contraception. Birth control pills don't prevent you from going through menopause—your eggs will still be dying off, and your estrogen and progesterone levels will stop fluctuating and drop to low menopausal levels. It just happens in the background so you may not really feel it. If you try going off the pill and find that you're still getting your period, you may wish to go back on it or try another hormonal treatment. But if you're in menopause, there's no need to use contraceptives anymore, and many of your perimenopausal symptoms will likely have dissipated. If you're still seeking relief, a different, targeted treatment may be a better option.

If you do decide to try birth control pills for contraception/perimenopausal symptoms, there are many, many different options, and you can work with your doctor to find the one that best suits you. It may seem redundant to have so many pills on the market since they all use the same overarching mechanism for quieting the reproductive system, but different formulations behave a little bit differently in the body, which influences potential side effects. Most birth control pills contain ethinyl estradiol and a progestin, of which there are a variety. Some progestins are slightly androgenic, meaning they have a male hormone–like quality that may make them a little more likely to cause acne. So those wouldn't be the pills for Nancy, Rebecca's patient whose pimples had returned with a vengeance during perimenopause. She was prescribed the birth control pill Yaz, which contains the progestin drospirenone, an anti-androgenic—and she stayed on it well into her fifties. Many other pills can provide desirable side effects, whether that's preventing acne or helping reduce water weight. But the effects vary based on the individual. It's possible for two women taking the same pill to have a completely different experience, so finding the right one can take a little trial and error.

One of the decisions you'll need to make when choosing a pill is whether you want to have a monthly period. Combined hormone pills come in three basic types: monophasic, biphasic, and triphasic, only one of which allows you to skip the bleeding. A monophasic pack, which is what most women prefer, provides the exact same dose of estrogen and progestin every day for 21 to 24 days, then 4 to 7 days of placebo pills. If you don't want to have a period, you can skip the placebos and just continue with the active ingredient pills. If you do skip your period, it's recommended that you take the active pills continuously for three months, then allow yourself to have a period to allow any built-up endometrial lining to shed and prevent unexpected spotting.

The other two types of pills, biphasic and triphasic, are synthesized in a way that varies the amount of estrogen and progestin from week to week, so they try to mimic the natural hormonal cycle more closely. But because these pills raise and lower hormone levels, the lining of your uterus will grow more similarly to a normal menstrual cycle, so you can't skip your period on these. We generally recommend monophasic pills for perimenopausal women. When you're dealing with hormone-related symptoms, you want to stop the hormonal ups and downs of the menstrual cycle, so mimicking the normal cycle isn't going to be as helpful. That said, varied-hormone pills can sometimes suit a woman better depending on the side effects and her symptoms.

There are a few other types of combined hormonal contraception available to you. One is a patch worn on the arm for three weeks (you change it once a week). It releases hormones into the bloodstream, where they do their job of preventing ovulation. On the fourth week, you don't wear a patch, and you get your period. You can also use the patch continuously (no "off" weeks) to skip having periods. Birth control rings are another option. You can insert the rings by yourself—no doctor visit needed. There are two different kinds of rings. One is the NuvaRing, which is inserted into your vagina and left in for three weeks, then removed for a week so you can get your period. After the period week is up, you put in a new one. (You can also skip this week off and insert a new ring immediately if you prefer.) The Annovera ring lasts a year; you just take it out for a week to menstruate, then put it back in. Both rings contain hormones that stop ovulation and thicken the mucus to stop sperm from advancing.

While combined hormonal birth control is a good choice for most perimenopausal women, some women are not candidates for any estrogen therapy. There are also times when the most common type of estrogen in combined hormonal birth control (called ethinyl estradiol) isn't the right estrogen to treat perimenopausal symptoms. The minipill, or progestin-only pill, as it's known, is estrogen free. Most contain the progestin norethindrone. It works well as a contraceptive and regulates the menstrual cycle, but it doesn't stop ovulation, so it is not likely to prevent the hormonal ups and downs of perimenopause. However, the minipill can potentially be combined with estradiol therapy for someone who wants to use a progestin-only form of contraception and is having perimenopausal symptoms such as moodiness, vaginal dryness, and night sweats that didn't resolve or lessen with therapies containing ethinyl estradiol.

There is also a newer progestin-only pill on the market that contains a different kind of progestin called drospirenone, which actually stops ovulation in the majority of users. We'll often prescribe it for women who haven't done well on, or can't take, combined hormone pills containing ethinyl estradiol, but who want to suppress the hormonal fluctuations that are contributing to their symptoms. We can also add in an estradiol patch if it makes sense for the patient. This combination works particularly well for women who haven't been able to control their hot flashes with other types of pills or if they have migraines with aura and can't take the traditional combined hormone pills with ethinyl estradiol.

Most women respond very well to combined hormonal birth control pills, but they don't always eliminate perimenopausal symptoms. If you're already on the pill and feeling symptoms similar to perimenopause, they could be what we call breakthrough symptoms. They're pretty rare for women on combined hormonal contraception, but they can happen, and we don't always know why. One possibility is that the pill they're on is too low-dose, or the type of estrogen it contains doesn't alleviate certain symptoms. We have different types of estrogen receptors throughout the body, from the uterus to the breasts to the liver, bone marrow, and the brain. Depending on the type of estrogen contained in a contraceptive pill, it may have more of a binding affinity for a particular receptor. It's possible—and this is conjecture—that one type of estrogen may have an affinity for brain receptors, so the pill with that type of estrogen works better on symptoms like brain fog, sleep, and hot flashes. Conversely, another type of estrogen doesn't have that brain-receptor affinity, so you get breakthrough symptoms. Ethinyl estradiol in particular doesn't work the same at the estrogen receptor as estradiol does, so it's possible to have or develop perimenopausal symptoms while taking a pill containing this type of estrogen. The bottom line here (and the reason we're taking the liberty of talking so much about all the different kinds) is that not all people react the same to different forms of estrogen. So if your first stab at a contraception-based remedy doesn't work, know that there are other options out there. Your doctor can help guide you through the trial-and-error process, hopefully hitting the target sooner rather than later.

Occasionally, what we'll also see is that, as women get closer to that final menstrual period—menopause—the pill they've long been taking just doesn't do it for them anymore. They're at a point where it might be best to switch to menopausal hormone therapy, which we'll talk about at length in the next chapter.

Intrauterine Devices (IUDs)

IUDs are small devices inserted into the uterus that work by preventing sperm from ever fertilizing an egg. While the modern IUD was developed in the twentieth century, inserting objects (paper, pebbles) into the uterus to prevent pregnancy dates back centuries. The precursor to the IUD used today was created in 1909, when a Polish doctor devised a flexible ring made of suturing silk and a tool to insert it. Although the device didn't go over very well—it prevented pregnancy but often caused infection—other inventors would seize on the general premise and develop variations over the next fifty years.

There are two types of IUDs available, one with hormones and one without. Both are made of plastic, shaped like a T, and have an inert string attached that aids in their removal. The nonhormonal version of the IUD uses copper to create an immune response in the uterus that creates a toxic environment for sperm. The "Copper T," or Paragard, lasts about ten years; the Miudella, a newer version of the nonhormonal IUD, currently has FDA approval for three years, but will likely be available for extended use as it garners subsequent approvals. Hormonal IUDs don't use copper; instead, they contain a reservoir along the stem of the T that contains the progestin levonorgestrel, which thickens cervical mucus and stops sperm in its tracks. Progestin-containing IUDs also cause thinning of the inside lining of the uterus, resulting in lighter, shorter periods, or no bleeding whatsoever. This type of device lasts three to eight years, depending on which brand you use.

Today, the IUD is the most popular form of birth control in the world—though not in the United States, due to the disaster of the Dalkon Shield. Prior to the Dalkon Shield's introduction in 1968, IUDs had become popular with American women thanks to the Lippes Loop, which was invented by a gynecologist names Jack Lippes and became the first safe, effective IUD on the market. The Dalkon Shield, however, was not particularly safe. Its shape made it painful to remove, and its string material made it easy for bacteria to move into the uterus and cause infections. The Dalkon Shield was taken off the market in 1974, and IUD use in the US plummeted. In the twenty-first century, however, the popularity of IUDs has steadily grown as more and more women are choosing them as a longer-term contraceptive. Contemporary IUDs are not only very safe but also one of the most effective forms of contraceptive out there.

The Dalkon Shield hit the market at a time when the FDA didn't closely monitor birth control devices. Now, IUDs are subject to strict FDA regulation, which means the manufacturers must demonstrate safety through extensive research and testing. The way contemporary devices are produced means the risk of infection is now very low, and, as noted, they're highly effective. Since IUDs only contain a progestin, no estrogen, they're a great option for women who don't want to or can't use combined hormonal contraception to manage the perimenopausal symptom of bleeding, and they can be combined with estradiol therapy to treat other symptoms. We also often recommend them to patients who have endometriosis or a lot of pain during their periods—progestin-containing IUDs can help with both.

Like birth control pills and any form of medication, IUDs do carry some risks. One that many patients ask about is breast cancer. A number of recent studies have found that IUDs can increase the risk of breast cancer, but only slightly. A recent study from Sweden found that there were 0.14 additional cases of breast cancer per 1,000 women. And to be honest, this wasn't a huge surprise—we have long known that there's a link between progestins (including those in birth control pills) and a small elevated risk for breast cancer. It's one of the factors we weigh when prescribing any medication or device that contains progestins. What was surprising, though, was that the Swedish study found that hormonal IUDs substantially reduced the risk of uterine and ovarian cancers. This exciting result just goes to show that there are pros and cons to every form of treatment.

We usually recommend hormonal IUDs for women in mid- to late perimenopause whose periods have become more irregular and the bleeding heavier. In about 99 percent of patients, the devices control bleeding very well because progestins stop the lining from growing. During perimenopause, estrogen can build up and stimulate growth in the uterine lining. This growth raises the risk of precancers and cancers. But the progestin in the hormonal IUDs keeps the interior of the uterus very thin, reducing bleeding significantly and helping prevent cancer. It can even stop bleeding entirely—about 70 percent of women get no bleeding at all. Note that these are effects from hormonal IUDs. Copper IUDs, on the other hand, can make periods heavier and crampier, so we don't generally prescribe them for women already having irregular and heavier bleeding. (The newer one may be less of a problem in this area, but we're still collecting data on that.)

Because hormonal IUDs contain only progestins, they don't counteract all perimenopausal symptoms. Occasionally, in the case of acne, they may even make them worse (levonorgestrel, for example, is a testosterone derivative, so it can cause an increase in androgenic effects like acne). You still ovulate with an IUD, so the roller coaster doesn't stop, and you may still experience hot flashes, brain fog, and mood symptoms. For women encountering those problems, we can add in an estrogen (estradiol) patch, much like we do when someone is on a progestin-only pill.

There are a couple of caveats here. Most hormonal IUDs contain 52 mg of levonorgestrel, but there are also some lower-dose IUDs out there. We know from research that, when combined with an estrogen patch, the 52 mg dose of progestin prevents the estrogen from bulking up the uterine lining to a hazardous thickness. But we don't know if the lower-dose IUD has enough progestin to counteract estrogen from a patch, so we don't recommend that particular duo. The other caveat is that we know the 52 mg hormonal IUDs work as birth control for eight years; but we don't know if the progestin levels stay high enough for eight years to counter the supplemental estrogen and prevent cancer. We only have data that shows it works for five years for this particular benefit, so if you're using it specifically as a menopausal hormone therapy in combination with estrogen and not just contraception, we recommend swapping it out at year five.

On a personal level, we both love IUDs for perimenopausal women. We've used them ourselves, and as it turns out, around 70 percent of ob-gyns choose IUDs for their own contraception. That's a pretty good endorsement.

Injections, Implants

Injections and implants are two other forms of contraception you may have used or heard of. While these work well for contraception, they're not as effective as birth control pills and IUDs for addressing perimenopausal symptoms, so we won't spend much time on them here.

The injectable form of birth control is called Depo-Provera, and the shots are given every three months. Depo-Provera (depot medroxyprogesterone acetate, or DMPA) is a type of progestin and works the way most progestins do, by thickening cervical mucus. If you are already using the Depo shot as your contraceptive and want to keep using it into perimenopause, it can easily be combined with an estrogen patch to calm perimenopausal symptoms, but we don't recommend women start the Depo shot in perimenopause because there are concerns that it accelerates bone loss with extended use. In a nineteen-year-old, that's not really a problem because they will regain bone when they come off it. But a forty-five-year-old doesn't have that luxury—the bone won't rebuild—so we tend not to prescribe it for women in midlife.

Implants are another type of contraception that, while excellent for birth control, are not a top choice for midlife women. The implant (Nexplanon) is about the size of a matchstick, and it is placed into your upper arm, where it will provide contraception for five years by slowly releasing a progestin into your system. As it happens, the progestin in implants both increases cervical mucus and stops eggs from leaving the ovaries, so it could theoretically be a good choice for women in peri-menopause. But it can also increase irregular bleeding. Perhaps that's one reason why it's not particularly popular with women in midlife. In any case, there's limited data on the use of Nexplanon combined with estradiol therapy to treat perimenopausal symptoms, so we don't rou-tinely use or recommend this combination.

It's quite possible that hormonal birth control will take you all the way up to and through menopause, easing your way so that symptoms are minimal and manageable. You may never need to think about menopausal hormone therapy. And if you do? We'll tell you all you need to know in the next chapter.

13

Menopausal Hormone Therapy

Resurrecting a Reputation

Hormone therapy goes the way of leeches.

—NATIONAL POST NEWSPAPER HEADLINE PREMATURELY PREDICTING
THE DEATH OF MENOPAUSAL HORMONE THERAPY, JULY 13, 2002

Menopausal hormone therapy (MHT) is a broad category of medicine that combines estrogen and progesterone to help counteract the many hormone-related symptoms of perimenopause and menopause. It was once called hormone replacement therapy, or HRT, but the name was gradually replaced with MHT to better reflect the fact that menopause is not a disease, and we are not trying to "replace" missing hormones to our premenopausal range. Because it's designed specifically for women in full menopause, MHT can be more effective at treating certain symptoms than birth control. But different forms of MHT, like the estradiol patch we mentioned in the last chapter, can be combined with contraceptives to provide broad coverage of both pregnancy prevention and symptom relief.

You have likely noticed that messages have been mixed about

hormone therapy over the last few decades. This roller coaster of coverage began on July 9, 2002, when representatives of the *Journal of the American Medical Association* (*JAMA*) called a press conference to report that a Women's Health Initiative (WHI) study investigating MHT, then better known as hormone replacement therapy, or HRT, had been abruptly halted after doctors determined that its health risks exceeded the benefits. It was headline news, and a bombshell for the medical community. Both of us remember exactly where we were at the time—Amy was in medical school at Mayo Clinic in Rochester, Minnesota, and the phones in the gynecology clinic were ringing off the hook with reporters wanting Mayo doctors to comment on the study. Over in Philadelphia, Rebecca was doing her residency. At the time, she was working in a clinic without many menopausal patients, but she happened to be sitting next to a menopause expert when they were told the news. She remembers the doctor responding with skepticism. "Where's the data?" she asked. "You can't just make a pronouncement like that without any data."

The lack of data—or more precisely, the misinterpretation of the data—was the crux of the issue, but that wouldn't be revealed until years later. In the immediate aftermath, many women stopped hormone therapy. A treatment that had been in regular use since as far back as the 1890s had suddenly been labeled "too risky." When the raw data from the study in question was finally released, it became clear that the risk of life-threatening side effects like cancer, blood clots, and dementia had been significantly overblown. The actual risks were incredibly rare and depended heavily on what age a woman started MHT. But the damage was done, as scores of women were now too afraid to ask their doctors for medications that could have benefited them greatly.

This was a shame, not only because hormone therapy can improve symptoms but also because it can help mitigate health risks. MHT has been shown to reduce the risk of heart attack and stroke in certain age groups; for women under sixty years old, or fewer than ten years from their final menstrual period, cardiovascular disease risk may decrease by up to 30 percent on MHT. It's believed this is because estrogen has a slightly anti-inflammatory effect on your blood vessels; when you have adequate estrogen in your system, the blood vessels stay relatively pliable and plaque-free. Women don't tend to develop significant cardiovascular disease until they run out of estrogen (notwithstanding genetic risk factors). So taking MHT might delay or even stop damage to the blood vessels that can lead to heart attack and stroke. However, if you start taking MHT after you've been in menopause for a while, it's likely that, without estrogen and due to the natural course of aging, your blood vessels have become less pliable and developed some plaque. Taking MHT at this stage can't undo those changes, and it may actually narrow vessels due to estrogen's mild clotting effect.

It's become clear that there's a "window of opportunity," a particular age range, where the benefits of MHT outweigh the risks. The current guidelines suggest it is safe to begin hormone therapy within five to ten years past your last period, or under age sixty. If you begin hormone therapy later than this, the cardiovascular risks may outweigh the benefits. You can safely stay on hormones after sixty, if you began taking them at a younger age. Of course, as with all rules, there are exceptions. One patient of Rebecca's, who was about ten and a half years out from her last period, was still having debilitating hot flashes, fifteen to twenty a day. Full-on night sweats prevented her from sleeping at night. "I can't live like this anymore," she said. She was given a full cardiovascular assessment—a stress test and an evaluation to see if there were calcium deposits in her arteries—and it showed that she was at very low risk for heart disease. In this case, and because she felt the risks were exceeded by the need to improve her patient's quality of life, Rebecca prescribed MHT. It resolved her patient's hot flashes, and her later test results showed no evidence of cardiovascular disease.

Like the pill, MHT can increase the risk of blood clots, but whether or not that risk should be a deciding factor in your treatment will depend on your age and health history. There's an increased risk of blood clots in all MHT users, regardless of age, when it's taken in pill form. If you've ever had a deep blood clot (thrombosis), have a clotting disorder, or cardiovascular disease, you would not be a candidate for MHT. For those who can take hormones, the risk seems to be lower if you receive the estrogen part of the combined hormone MHT through the skin via patch, gel, or spray or via the vagina in the form of a vaginal ring.

Like cardiac disease, MHT has been linked to both higher and lower risks of dementia, depending on when you start the therapy. Data from the WHI and other studies shows an increased risk of dementia from MHT in patients who start hormonal therapy over the age of sixty. This is likely related to vascular changes in the brain: like your blood vessels, your brain can develop plaques as you age, which can be a precursor to dementia. However, population-based studies show that, in women who start MHT during perimenopause or early menopause, there is no increase in dementia later in life—though there is no decrease either. An exception to this is in women who experience premature menopause (before age forty-five) and are using MHT at least until the "natural" age of menopause, about fifty-one. In these women, hormonal therapy can actually help protect against the development of dementia later in life. (Why exactly is not known, as we don't see dementia protection in women who go through menopause at a normal age. This part needs more study.)

MHT can also be enormously helpful in helping maintain bone density. Bone protection, along with hot flashes, genitourinary symptoms, and premature estrogen deficiency, is one of the main FDA-approved uses for MHT. You can benefit from MHT's bone-strengthening effects no matter when you start taking it, but unfortunately that benefit goes away once you stop taking MHT. One of the many negative impacts of the inaccurate reporting on the 2002 study is that many women who decided not to take MHT due to scary news reports are now seeing worse effects of osteoporosis than they might have if they'd taken MHT, not to mention the quality of life benefits they may have been able to take advantage of had the study been more carefully presented.

Other benefits of MHT include a lower incidence of diabetes and certain cancers. Women taking MHT have reduced risk of developing type 2 diabetes (17 to 30 percent, depending on the study), especially if they have a predisposition such as prediabetes, metabolic syndrome, or polycystic ovarian syndrome. Many studies also suggest an association between MHT and a small reduced incidence of colorectal cancer (though other studies do not confirm this finding) as long as you are on MHT, though unfortunately, like the bone health benefits, this effect only lasts as long as you're taking MHT and goes away when you stop.

Because it's a hormonal treatment, MHT does have some effect on your likelihood to develop hormone-influenced cancers. Like combined hormone birth control, combined estrogen and progesterone MHT significantly lowers the risk of endometrial cancer by ensuring there's no uncontrolled growth in the uterine lining, but estrogen alone without progesterone can actually increase your risk. Ovarian cancer risk is less clear—observational studies have shown a small statistically significant increased risk of ovarian cancer in women using both estrogen alone and combined estrogen and progesterone, but in the WHI study, there was no increased risk of ovarian cancer with combined estrogen and progesterone use. The big question many women have— and the scariest part of the misleading 2002 press release—has to do with the risk of breast cancer.

Among the worrisome takeaways from the misleading reports about the WHI study was that HRT was linked to a very high risk of breast cancer. While reported in the media as a 20 percent risk increase (an interpretation of the relative risk of 1.2), in actuality, we now know that the increased risk of breast cancer for combined estrogen and progesterone use is nine women per ten thousand. This is less than the increased risk that comes from drinking two glasses of wine a night and having dense breast tissue, and similar to the risk of obesity and low physical activity. The risk may also be lower for women taking micronized progesterone intermittently and who start MHT early. In women taking estrogen-only MHT, the risk of breast cancer does not rise and may even decrease. Most importantly, in the eighteen-year follow-up of both arms of the WHI study, there were, significantly, no increased deaths from breast cancer in any of the groups studied. Any breast cancers that were found in the women under study were early-stage and curable. So the risk isn't nothing, but like many other medications, it's important to weigh them against the health and quality of life benefits.

WHEN MHT SHOULD *NOT* BE USED

IF YOU HAVE ANY OF THE FOLLOWING MEDICAL COMPLICATIONS, MHT IS NOT A FIT FOR YOU:

- Pregnancy

- Unexplained vaginal bleeding

- Liver disease

- History of deep venous thrombosis or pulmonary embolism (blood clots), known clotting disorders

- History of coronary heart disease, stroke, or ministroke

- Untreated hypertension (if your blood pressure is well controlled, it's fine to use MHT)

- History of estrogen-dependent cancer (such as breast, some uterine and ovarian)

Making Sense of the Choices

The menopausal transition is a continuum, so there's no exact time when MHT is the best option. As a general rule, we recommend considering MHT as you get closer to menopause, since it can often be a better option than birth control or other perimenopausal interventions for comprehensively controlling the symptoms that tend to escalate in menopause rather than abate, like hot flashes, poor sleep, vaginal dryness, and incontinence. When you're on the perimenopause/menopause borderline, you may still be getting a period but find that menopausal symptoms are affecting you more so than the hormonal ups and downs of perimenopause. This is where MHT can be helpful. Plus, with menopause at your doorstep, you've likely reached the point where you may want to begin addressing age-related issues like cardiovascular disease and osteoporosis, which, as outlined, MHT can help with.

If menopause is still a ways off (an assessment your doctor can help make), MHT may not be the best option. Also remember, you don't *need* to take MHT (this is why we no longer call it "hormone replacement," which suggests a disorder that requires replacing). Plenty of women live long, healthy lives with manageable menopausal symptoms and no bone or cardiovascular disease without the support of MHT. This is what your doctor is there for; to help you make the right call. Just remember that if you do decide to start MHT, you'll want to do so within ten years (more or less) of your period stopping completely in order to avoid the risks and reap the benefits.

MHT Options

The way we typically prescribe menopausal hormone therapy is by combining estradiol, a synthesized form of estrogen molecularly identical to what the body produces naturally, with a progesterone pill. The progesterone is also molecularly identical to the human-made form.

We prefer these types of estrogen and progesterone because they have the fewest side effects and seem to work well for most people.

Whenever possible, we like to prescribe estradiol in transdermal—through the skin—forms. Estradiol taken orally has to go through the liver before dispersing in the body. The liver makes proteins called clotting factors that help the blood to clot. As estradiol passes through, it increases the formation of these clotting factors, thus increasing the risk of blood clots. Non-oral estradiol, on the other hand, has minimal contact with the liver and thus little impact on the formation of clotting factors. Transdermal methods are usually easy to use. The most common of the transdermal estradiol delivery systems is the patch. Some versions of the patch are changed once a week, but we prefer the ones that get changed twice a week because they're smaller and the adhesive seems to work better and is less irritating to the skin. Transdermal estradiol is also available in a spray and in a gel, but the gel can be irritating over time, especially to already-dry perimenopausal skin, but they all work to get estrogen into your body and mitigate symptoms.

HORMONE SOURCES

You may wonder—where do the hormones in MHT come from? There is a version of estrogen made from pregnant-mare urine—conjugated equine estrogen (CEE)—but other than that, all estrogens on the market, as well as progestins and progesterone—are made synthetically in a lab and have been since the 1970s. By synthetically we mean that molecules from various compounds are stitched together to create another compound that has the same molecular structure as the desired hormone. When people talk about bioidentical (sometimes called body identical) hormones, what they're referring to are hormones made in a lab with ingredients that are molecularly identical to the ones the body makes. But so are the hormones used in conventional

MHT formulations. Except for CEE, they're *all* molecularly identical to the real things; none are "natural."

What sets conventional, FDA-approved hormones apart from the ones marketed as bioidentical is that they're calibrated into standardized amounts, just like an aspirin you might get from the pharmacy. Bioidentical hormones, by contrast, are measured and combined by compounding pharmacists. That makes it sound like you're getting a special, customized version of MHT, but when patients inquire about bioidentical hormones, we always emphasize that the compounding pharmacist making the medication isn't creating a special mix just for you. Compounded bioidentical hormones offer no special benefit or difference in terms of tailoring and in fact may be less safe or effective than FDA-approved medications.

Adding the term "natural" to a medication can give it a misleading halo, even if it is truly natural, like the hormone conjugated equine estrogen. We both limit the use of CEE on ethical grounds. The mares used to make the hormone are kept continually pregnant because it's the only time they make CEE. The horses are housed in a corral with a urine catheter inserted twenty-three hours a day and are only allowed to move around for about an hour. The results of all those pregnancies, the foals, sometimes eventually become CEE sources themselves. Others are used for dog food or racing. Overall, we strongly recommend using the synthetic, lab-made hormones in FDA-approved medications or using nonhormonal therapies if the idea of synthetic hormones makes you uncomfortable.

Another way to get estradiol is through a vaginal ring. There's a specific kind of low-dose ring that is used as a localized treatment of vaginal dryness, but here we're talking about a slightly higher-dose estradiol ring that is used for a broader range of menopausal symptoms. The ring releases estrogen transdermally through the skin of the vagina and systemically. It lasts three months, and you just change it out yourself. It's very convenient and doesn't impact the liver like oral estrogens can. Unfortunately, the ring is often not covered by insurance.

Progesterone can also be used to help manage perimenopause symptoms like difficulty sleeping and irregular bleeding either alone or in conjunction with estradiol, although it is almost always paired with estrogen. This works in a similar way to progestin-only birth control but is dosed differently to help specifically target perimenopause and menopause symptoms. While estradiol can be taken in a few different forms, progesterone must be taken orally, since the molecule is too big to be absorbed through the skin. It comes in a micronized pill form, which means that it's suspended in oil, which enhances uptake into your system. Progesterone should never, ever be compounded into a topical form because if you take it out of that micronized form it really doesn't absorb very well. (Although a vaginal version of natural progesterone does exist, it's dosed for fertility and not recommended for treating the menopausal transition.) The progesterone pill is best taken at night so that it can work to soothe the brain and help you sleep more deeply.

Although micronized progesterone is our preferred progestogen (progesterone-like compound), another class of progestogens, called progestins, can also be used. These are a large class of synthetic molecules, based on progesterone but adapted to be slightly better absorbed. These are sometimes the same as those found in birth control methods. We may choose to use a progestin if a patient has irregular bleeding on micronized progesterone. There are also some progestins that can work as birth control and suppress ovulation while also protecting the endometrium from growing too "fluffy" from estradiol therapy.

Like birth control, there are other forms of MHT that offer a combination of hormones. These contain an estrogen and either micronized progesterone or a progestin. The micronized progesterone products are oral while the progestin-containing options can be in a patch or oral form. Other combination products resemble an ultra-low-dose birth control pill. They're actually packaged in packs like birth control pills and contain hormones that you would typically see in birth control, such as ethinyl estradiol and progestins. Depending on your symptoms and other treatment paths you may be pursuing, these can work well.

Ending MHT

While age is an important factor in starting MHT, there's no specific recommendations for how old you should be when you go off it. In general, if you've been taking them since menopause onset, you can usually keep taking them indefinitely unless your risk factors change. Many people mistakenly think they must stop at a certain age, but by taking estrogen through the years, you have likely prevented those changes in your vascular system that might otherwise cause a blood clot–plaque pileup if you had started hormones at a later date. We tell our patients that the only reason they need to stop MHT is if they develop breast cancer, dementia, cardiovascular disease, or blood clots. But absent that, staying on hormones because they make you feel good and are helping to protect your long-term health are perfectly acceptable reasons to continue.

If you want to stop taking the medication, our recommendation for when to go off it usually depends on the main symptoms you initially wanted to treat. The patient who primarily went on MHT for hot flashes and doesn't want to continue will generally taper down at year seven or ten to see if her hot flashes are gone. If they are, she can go off the hormones. A second type of patient, one who was using MHT to deal with brain fog and sleep issues, might choose to take hormones until she retires so she can continue to function at a high level while working. She can taper off MHT when ready.

And, as noted, if you want to keep taking it forever, you often can. A study published in the journal *Menopause* in 2024 looked at the records of 10 million female Medicare recipients and found that, compared with women who never used or discontinued use of MHT before age sixty-five, women who stayed on MHT past the age of sixty-five had significant risk reductions in mortality, breast cancer, lung cancer, colorectal cancer, and cardiovascular events. There was a slight increase in breast cancer risk, so that's something that needs to be taken into consideration when making the decision to stay on hormones long-term.

MHT can be a great overall solution to symptoms during perimenopause and into menopause, and it can also be used in conjunction with other medications to combat specific symptoms, such as using an estradiol patch to deal with hot flashes while taking a progestin-only birth control. If you only have a few specific symptoms, you may want to try targeting those more directly, but if you're experiencing a whole range of perimenopausal issues and think a hormonal remedy might be for you, or you're looking to come off birth control and want to try a hormonal treatment that you can keep taking into older age, MHT can be a great choice.

14

Everything Else

Nonhormonal Treatments

Pharmaceutical companies seem to have suddenly realized there
are women over fifty-five who need medications (and who have the
buying power to purchase them).

—RESEARCH PHYSICIAN

Andrea is a patient who isn't anti-hormones per se, but she is
someone who doesn't tolerate most medications well. "I'm the
kind of person who gets every side effect you can get from drugs," she
told Amy. She had, for instance, tried taking birth control pills for her
late-perimenopausal symptoms—she was in the throes of hot flashes,
blue moods, and middle-of-the-night awakenings—and that hadn't
gone great. And given her side-effect issues, she was too nervous to try
MHT. "That's okay," Amy told her. "We have other options." As Amy
took Andrea through the list of nonhormonal treatments, Andrea
stopped her at hypnotherapy. It appealed to her.

A few weeks later, Andrea came back and reported that the hypnosis had been fascinating—and it improved her symptoms. Her lifelong anxiety, which had ramped up during perimenopause, was better. Her mood was better. Her sleep was better. Her hot flashes were still coming on, but because she was sleeping well and her mood was improved, she could handle them (and she got a ChiliPad, which helped, too).

There's a lot of evidence to suggest that hormone-based therapies offer the most effective comprehensive relief from perimenopausal symptoms. But they're not the only solutions available, and plenty of women seek out nonhormonal options, whether because they have a personal history of breast cancer, cardiovascular disease, blood clots, or stroke, or perhaps because they may have used hormonal therapy in the past, and it didn't work well. Or, like Andrea, they had side effects that were intolerable. Or maybe it's just that their symptoms aren't that bad, and they'd prefer to seek out other options before taking medication.

Most nonhormonal treatments, it should be noted, don't get to the root cause of many symptoms—they can't help with hormone volatility or diminishment. Nonetheless, many patients have success with them, and in consultations, we offer them as options to all our patients whether they're hormone-averse or not. What follows is a rundown of those treatments that have some data behind them indicating that they may solve an array of perimenopausal symptoms. A lot of the data focuses on hot flashes because that's easy to measure, but we've tried to include here those nonhormonal remedies that seem to hit several targets, even if there's less clinical research regarding sleep, brain fog, or other harder-to-measure symptoms. And of course, just because a treatment doesn't have data behind it doesn't necessarily mean that it won't work. It just means it's harder to predict what your personal outcome might be.

Supplements

It's not easy to find supplements that can have a comprehensive effect on perimenopausal symptoms, but there are two that have a little data behind them. One is purified cytoplasm of pollen (PCP), a dietary supplement available primarily in Europe and North America under several brand names. It contains two active ingredients: a pure pollen extract and a blend of a pollen and extract of flower pistil (fittingly, the ovary part of a flower). Observational studies suggest PCP reduces hot flashes, muscle aches, sleep disturbances, and mood symptoms. But a review of studies also showed no difference in perimenopausal and menopausal symptoms when control groups were utilized, suggesting a strong placebo effect. It's safe, though, so perhaps worth a shot.

A second supplement that may offer some comprehensive relief is ammonium succinate. Often sold under the brand name Amberen, ammonium succinate has been studied in two small randomized, placebo-controlled trials. An analysis of the data indicated that it reduced a number of symptoms, including hot flashes, sadness and irritability, and difficulty sleeping. The studies also showed an increase in blood estradiol levels. Given the limited data and the fact that both studies were sponsored by the manufacturer, its efficacy is uncertain, but we've had a few patients try it and report some success.

When considering supplements, remember this: Supplements in the United States are 100 percent unregulated by the FDA, and there have been some reports of people getting lead poisoning from herbal medications they bought on the internet. Some supplements, when tested, also turn out to have pharmaceuticals or hormones in them that aren't listed on the label. Certain supplements, because they're billed as an extract of something found in the wild, can seem innocuous, but manufacturers will often add other ingredients to the formulation, including estrogens, so you want to be careful. You don't know what you may potentially be exposed to. They're also not routinely tested for accuracy, so it's possible they may not contain any of what is indicated on the label. If you want to try an herbal remedy, stay on the beaten path, buying from reputable stores and choosing brands or specific supplements that have been independently verified, indicating that they've been made using good manufacturing processes. Look for these indicators on the label: "nonprofit US Pharmacopoeia (USP) Dietary Supplement Verification Program" or "ConsumerLab.com."

Nonprescription Medical Interventions

Because so many women either can't take hormones or choose not to, there's been an increased focus on medical interventions beyond medication that can offer perimenopausal and menopausal symptom relief. And it turns out, some of them work very well. There are three that we typically talk about with patients. One is hypnotherapy (also called clinical hypnosis) of the sort that Andrea, Amy's patient, tried for her perimenopausal symptoms. During hypnosis, the brain switches into a state that not only makes it more open to suggestion but also affects autonomic functions like heart rate, blood flow, and breathing. As you might expect, hypnosis primarily impacts symptoms originating in the brain: While the mechanism isn't entirely clear, a few studies have shown that hypnosis can be effective for hot flashes, anxiety, and poor sleep. In 2024, the Menopause Society also did a review of eight hypnotherapy studies and found that hypnotherapy significantly lowered hot flash frequency and severity and improved quality of life, sleep quality, and mood by 60 percent.

The Menopause Society review also compared hypnotherapy to fifteen cognitive behavioral therapy (CBT) studies. We've talked about CBT as a remedy for insomnia and for mood issues like depression and anxiety, but CBT can be tailored to treat various symptoms, and several studies have shown that it can help improve hot flashes, night sweats, depressive mood, insomnia, stress, anxiety, and sexual issues. And while the researchers found that hypnotherapy had better results than CBT, especially in regard to hot flashes, they did find that CBT was helpful in reducing the daily disruptions and angst associated with hot flashes.

In 2024, Korean researchers published a small study testing out the effect of CBT developed specifically for perimenopausal women and comparing it to what the researchers termed "treatment-as-usual" (gynecologist-provided education about symptoms, lifestyle advice, and MHT as needed). Forty women, ages forty to sixty, completed the study, which involved an hour-long CBT session per week for eight weeks. As compared to the usual treatment group, the CBT women had more improvement in emotional symptoms, anxiety, and overall quality of life.

How cognitive behavioral therapy works is less of a mystery than hypnosis. It doesn't make certain symptoms like hot flashes go away altogether, but as the Menopause Society study found, it just helps you cope better. When you worry about symptoms, it sets up a cycle where you may obsess over them, making them even worse as well as heightening your stress and anxiety about the hot flashes. CBT can make all that nonstop thinking about the possibility of having a hot flash (or other symptoms) go away.

Another medical intervention, called a stellate ganglion block, is a little more invasive than hypnotherapy or CBT but has been effective in treating a number of perimenopausal symptoms, including hot flashes, sleep difficulties, and even incontinence. The procedure is usually administered by specialists at a pain clinic and involves having an injection in the front side of your neck aimed at a "ball" of neurons that reside there. The injection blocks signals from the sympathetic nervous system (which controls your fight-or-flight reactions, including heart and breathing rates) and has been used to remedy various types of pain and heart conditions. The stellate ganglion block has even been used off-label to treat post-traumatic stress disorder (PTSD).

Nonhormonal Prescription Medications

As much as we'd like to say there's a single magic perimenopausal bullet that makes every symptom go away, it's usually more of a whack-a-mole situation: You may need a combination of remedies to tame the symptoms well enough to make you feel like yourself again. This can mean "layering" remedies that are hormone-based (say, an estrogen patch and an IUD) with nonhormonal solutions, including nonhormonal prescription medications.

For example, Carla is a patient of Amy's who was encountering hot flashes, night sweats, brain fog, insomnia, joint pain, really bad depression, and anxiety—almost every perimenopausal symptom you can imagine. She hadn't tolerated the progestins in birth control pills very well in the past, so that wasn't a treatment option. Instead, Carla left Amy's office with an IUD (for birth control and bleeding control) as well as a prescription for an estrogen patch (for treating the symptoms the IUD wouldn't cover).

These treatments helped with a lot of her symptoms, but she was still struggling with insomnia. Amy added a prescription for gabapentin, a nonhormonal medication that's typically used for nerve-related pain and seizures but, at much lower doses, has also been shown to improve hot flashes. Because it has a sedating effect, it can improve sleep as well. You might remember that earlier in the book we talked about the body's GABA (gamma-aminobutyric acid) system, which blocks certain neurons from communicating. In the case of neurons that communicate pain as well as stress and anxiety, this can be beneficial. Gabapentin, the drug, mimics the GABA system's message-blocking ability and, in that way, can interfere with the neural dispatches that trigger wakefulness, hot flashes, and other perimenopausal symptoms. It's a medication that many doctors keep in their symptom-relief toolbox, though patience on the part of patients is required: It may take six to twelve weeks before all its benefits kick in. For Carla, gabapentin turned out to be the perfect solution. She began nodding off easily and sleeping through the night. It took layering three types of therapy, but she ultimately was able to substantially improve her quality of life.

Layering is a common way to approach comprehensive care without using hormones. If you come in with hot flashes and some depression, your best option may be Veozah for the flashing (see pages 167–68) and an antidepressant. If you also have incontinence, your doctor may add in oxybutynin, a drug typically used for overactive bladder. If you're experiencing insomnia, maybe a gabapentin prescription is in order. Talk to your doctor about all your symptoms so you can get the best possible treatment protocol.

Part Four

Next Steps

Menopause and Lifelong Wellness

15

Cardiovascular Health

Your Heart Needs Love and Attention

Around the time she turned fifty, Elizabeth visited her primary care physician for the physical she'd been putting off for several years. When she got the results of her blood panel back, she was alarmed. She'd never seen her cholesterol numbers so high. What had happened in the intervening years? Only one thing she could think of: menopause. Before she even had time to discuss the results with her doctor, Elizabeth made an appointment with Amy, seeking a prescription for menopausal hormone therapy. "My cholesterol is really high right now because of menopause," she said, adding, "I need estrogen to make it go down."

Elizabeth wasn't entirely right about menopause being the cause of her rising low-density lipoprotein cholesterol. But she wasn't entirely wrong either. Research that follows women throughout the menopausal transition shows that cholesterol and other lipids do rise in the late stages of the transition. And loss of estrogen is considered a contributing factor to the higher lipids and what they indicate—increased risk of cardiovascular disease. But it's only a tiny piece of a much more complex picture.

Heart health can become an issue in midlife for many reasons, including familial and lifestyle factors, as well as the effects of aging. So it's not so much that the menopausal transition *causes* increased cardiovascular risk as it is that it *coincides* with a time of life when the heart and blood vessels become more vulnerable. Which is why now is the perfect time to focus on what you can do to protect yourself from cardiovascular disease, the number one cause of death in women.

In our experience, few women in midlife worry much about cardiovascular disease, an umbrella term for many heart- and vascular-related conditions, including coronary heart disease and stroke. Instead, their fears tend to be focused on breast cancer—not a risk we should ignore, but one that is far less likely to occur than a heart-related problem. Cardiovascular disease, in fact, kills more women than all forms of cancer combined (this is true for most races and ethnic groups, except Asian American, Pacific Islander, and Hispanic people—for these groups heart disease is second to cancer). If you didn't know that, you're not alone. When the American Heart Association did a survey on women's awareness of heart disease, the organization found that only 44 percent of women knew that it's the leading cause of death. Luckily, there are a lot of ways to protect yourself from heart attack, stroke, and other related conditions, especially if you begin these strategies during your perimenopausal years.

Why Risk Increases Now

Cardiovascular disease is not only the number one cause of death for women; it's the number one cause of death for men, too. However, there are some differences in the level of risk. Men's likelihood of dying from cardiovascular-related causes is always greater than women's, and the risk begins to rise when men are in their late forties. Women's risk begins to rise with age as well, but not until women are in their fifties and sixties. Then, when women reach their late sixties and seventies, they begin to catch up with men, and the gap between the sexes narrows. (In regard to other causes of death, men and women are mostly neck and neck, though men are always at somewhat higher risk of dying from any cause.)

Aging across the sexes is associated with various changes in the heart and blood vessels. For instance, over time, the walls of the heart may thicken so it holds less blood and becomes less efficient at beating when it's taxed by exercise or stress. The valves of the heart, which control blood flow, become stiffer, as do the blood vessels. Stiffness in the blood vessels makes them more prone to plaque buildup, raising the risk of blockages that cause heart attack or stroke. But women, unlike men, are protected from these changes a little longer due to the effects of estrogen.

One of the factors underlying cardiovascular disease is inflammation. In some cases, inflammation acts as a protective mechanism, like the swelling that results when you sprain your ankle. But it can also interfere with the body's normal operation. Estrogen, one of many chemicals in the body that have anti-inflammatory properties, helps prevent damage caused by inflammation. In the cardiovascular system, estrogen prevents plaque from clogging the arteries. But as estrogen diminishes over the course of the menopausal transition, the body's ability to deter plaque also diminishes, leading to a rise in cardiovascular risk. This is also why MHT has some positive cardiac effects for women when started in perimenopause or early menopause.

HOT FLASH OR HEART ATTACK?

Your heart is racing. Or you're having heart palpitations and chest pain. Or both. Does this mean you're having a heart attack? During perimenopause it's common for scary heart symptoms to occur. Sometimes it's a hot flash or anxiety, but it's never a bad idea to get an evaluation (especially if you have chest pain), because these symp-toms, even smack-dab in the middle of perimenopause, can be a sign of an abnormal heart rhythm or other heart-related problem. And although it's less common than in older women, you can still have a heart attack in your forties, so it's good to double-check.

Heart attacks, when they do happen, tend to present differently in women and men, in part because the two sexes develop plaque a little differently. Men tend to get plaque in their larger cardiac blood vessels, whereas women tend to see more plaque in their smaller blood vessels, downstream. Blood vessels are like branching trees, with big branches toward the center of the body, then smaller branches coming off these, and then the tiny little branches at the end. Women get more tiny vessel disease, and, for this reason, their heart attack symptoms are often more subtle.

Men may describe heart attacks as crushing chest pain; women often get neck pain, a little bit of pain in the upper arm, and pain on the left side of the chest. They also get nausea and sweating—something you might also experience during a hot flash—or sometimes feel like they're having heartburn. If you're having heart attack symptoms or any kind of cardiac issue, it's important to get checked out, just in case.

Reducing Risk

Heart and blood vessel health is influenced by many factors. A genetic history of high cholesterol or other cardiovascular issues, or environmental factors like tobacco exposure, can raise your risk. Likewise, cardiovascular issues that might have appeared during pregnancy, like high blood pressure or gestational diabetes, can indicate a higher risk for later developing cardiovascular disease. But unlike many other diseases, there are a lot of things you can do to lower your risk to mitigate these uncontrollable factors.

Eliminating Smoking, Reducing Drinking

Smoking is one of the worst things you can do for your heart health. While many people think of smoking as a danger to the lungs, it can have a cascade of effects across the whole body. The lungs act as a gateway to the cardiovascular system, where blood can pick up the chemicals you've inhaled and disperse them throughout the body. And it's these chemicals that damage the cardiovascular system, thickening and narrowing the blood vessels, helping to build up plaque, lowering HDL ("good") cholesterol, raising triglycerides, and causing other negative effects.

Smoking can also make blood sticky and more likely to clot, and vaping is no less risky than cigarettes. Vaping pens contain nicotine that adversely affects the blood vessels and other chemicals that can be harmful, too. Observational studies have also linked frequent marijuana smoking to increased incidence of heart attack and stroke. And while we're on the topic of mood-altering substances, we'd be remiss if we didn't say something about alcohol. We'll discuss alcohol more in the next chapter, but when it comes to cardiovascular health, even modest consumption of alcohol can raise both blood pressure levels and triglycerides (one of the harmful lipids).

Eating Well

In general, a healthy diet is important for perimenopausal women, especially as you manage the natural weight gain that comes at this time. When it comes to heart health specifically, you can make a difference in your level of risk by maximizing your intake of healthy foods and minimizing your intake of foods that are known to raise cholesterol and triglycerides. Studies have shown that the most heart-healthy diet is high in fruits, vegetables, whole grains, legumes, and nuts, and low in red and processed meats and sugary foods. Regardless of what specific diet a person adheres to—a Mediterranean-style diet, a plant-based diet, the DASH diet, or just simple good nutrition—eating in this way leads to a 14 to 21 percent reduction in cardiovascular risk.

These types of diets are typically rich in potassium, fiber, calcium, and magnesium, all of which help lower blood pressure. And they leave little room on the plate for foods high in sodium, which often increases blood pressure. High blood pressure (or hypertension) refers to the phenomenon of blood—as it's pumped out of your heart—being forceful enough to strain and damage your blood vessels. The process of repairing that damage can lead to plaque and its associated risks, like heart attack or stroke. Some research also suggests sodium can increase inflammation.

A nutritious plate also leaves little room for foods rich in saturated fat, a fat mostly found in red meat and dairy products and known to raise LDL cholesterol levels. LDLs (low-density lipoproteins) are considered the "bad" kind of cholesterol because they contribute to the buildup of plaque, similarly contributing to your risk of a blockage or cardiac event.

While it's important to limit saturated fats, fat in general isn't bad. Some fats—including the monounsaturated fats found in olive oil; avocado, peanut, canola, high-oleic safflower, and sunflower oils; avocados; and most nuts—can improve heart health. Likewise, some polyunsaturated fats, especially omega-3 fatty acids, can improve cholesterol levels by raising your level of HDLs (high-density lipoproteins), which help cholesterol move from the cardiovascular system back to the liver. Fatty fish like salmon, mackerel, and sardines, flaxseeds, walnuts, canola oil, and un-hydrogenated soybean oil are all good sources of these fats.

Exercising Often

Exercise isn't just important for weight management and bone health. Cardiovascular exercise, as the name indicates, is an important component of reducing risk of cardiovascular disease. Cardio (aerobic) exercise includes anything that gets your heart rate up and makes you sweat for an extended period of time (and isn't a hot flash!), strengthens the heart, and helps keep resting blood pressure and heart rate low, reducing strain on the system. But one of the things that's so critical about exercise is that it increases HDL cholesterol levels. This is the type of cholesterol that carries the bad cholesterol, LDL, out of the arteries. You want a high HDL cholesterol count, and exercise is one of the few ways to get it.

The American Heart Association recommends doing at least 150 minutes of moderate-intensity aerobic exercise per week, or 75 minutes of vigorous aerobic exercise, or a combination of the two. The organization also recommends strength training two times a week. You already know that strength training can circumvent some of the muscle and bone loss that begins to ramp up during the menopausal transition (see page 126). Research also suggests that by improving lipids, blood pressure, and blood vessel health, physical activity can also lower the risk of heart disease by 17 percent. An exercise program that combines cardio and strength training is one of the best ways to maintain good health through perimenopause and beyond.

Conditions That Increase Risk

Sometimes cardiovascular disease is considered a condition unto itself, but there are a number of conditions that can significantly increase your risk of cardiac issues. Top among those precursor conditions is diabetes. High blood sugar, a hallmark of diabetes, can injure blood vessels and the nerves that control the heart. As a result, people with diabetes (especially type 2 diabetes) are twice as likely to have heart disease or stroke as people without diabetes. Cardiovascular disease is the cause of death for two-thirds of diabetics, but you can limit your risk by ensuring your diabetes is well controlled and your blood sugar is kept at a steady level. Controlling diabetes is important no matter how old you are, but it becomes even more essential during midlife, when age starts to increase risk as well.

Obesity is another condition that can contribute to heart disease, though your risk may depend more on your body composition than your actual weight. Not all overweight people are destined to have cardiovascular issues, and some research indicates that in women, heart disease is much more related to how much muscle versus how much fat you have. In other words, even if you're overweight to the point of obesity, having a lot of muscle seems to be protective—another reason to integrate strength training into your routine.

While being overweight can contribute to potential risk, the number on the scale is less important than keeping an eye out for key warning signs of potential cardiovascular issues: high lipid levels, diabetes, high blood pressure, and/or sleep apnea. Sleep apnea, as discussed in chapter 4, can cause irregular heartbeats, endangering the cardiovascular system. The disorder also disrupts sleep so that your heart doesn't get the recovery time it needs to maintain optimal health. These threats to the cardiovascular system are serious: Sleep apnea increases the risk of heart failure by 140 percent and the risk of coronary heart disease by 30 percent.

Monitoring Risk

The best way to stay on top of your cardiovascular health is to have your blood pressure checked every year and your lipid levels checked at an interval determined by your physician. By lipids we mean cholesterol—LDL, HDL, and total cholesterol—triglycerides and lipoprotein (a), or Lp(a). Each of these factors impacts your cardiovascular system in different ways. Triglycerides, for instance, are an acute, reactive measure of how your blood reacts to food. If you eat macaroni and cheese the night before your triglycerides are tested, they'll likely be up. If you're eating foods with healthier monounsaturated fats or omega-3 fatty acids, your triglycerides may go down. Lp(a) is similar to LDL cholesterol in that it can cause plaque buildup and other problems that may lead to clotting or a rupture of blood vessels. It's also used as a marker for the amount of inflammation in the vessels and can be an important predictor of cardiovascular disease, so it's important to get it checked regularly.

We also recommend regular hemoglobin A1C tests, which can show your average blood sugar level over the previous two to three months. The test is one of the tools for diagnosing diabetes and other metabolic disorders that can ultimately affect the heart. It lets your doctor get an idea of how the insulin part of your system is working, so even if your lipid numbers are great, you'll know that there may still be a risk from a diabetes standpoint.

Your primary care physician and even your gynecologist can order these tests for you—you don't need to go to a cardiologist. But if your lipid panel plus other factors—such as the hemoglobin A1C test results, having a family history and/or, say, a history of gestational diabetes—combine to leave you at very high risk of cardiovascular disease, your physician should then recommend that you see a cardiologist. A cardiologist can run tests, like an electrocardiogram (EKG), stress test, and/or a cardiac calcium test, to further investigate your risk.

If it's just a matter of elevated lipids, that may be something your regular doctor can help you address, first by helping you map out lifestyle changes, then by prescribing medication if necessary. The most commonly prescribed medication for high cholesterol is a statin, a class of drugs that discourage the production of cholesterol in the liver and help remove it from the bloodstream. Studies show that statins lower the risk not only of death due to cardiovascular disease but death from all causes, and specifically in women. In women, statins also lower the risk of heart attack. There are other types of drugs that can be prescribed for high cholesterol, but statins are well studied and are the ones that most people seem to tolerate best.

So what happened to Elizabeth, Amy's patient, and her request for menopausal hormone therapy to benefit her heart health? Ultimately, she ended up starting MHT and taking a low-dose statin. Estrogen is not a cure-all for high cholesterol, and Elizabeth's elevated lipids were likely caused by a variety of factors, but supplemental estrogen can still be helpful for general cardiac health. Studies have shown a cardio-protective effect with long-term use of conjugated equine estrogens in women who start MHT at the transition to menopause. We really don't have as much data on the protective effects of estradiol, but we do know that oral estradiol has more of a positive impact on choles-terol than transdermal estradiol because it passes through the liver, the site of cholesterol production. Is it enough to counter the higher risk of clotting created by oral estradiol? If you're considering MHT for cardiovascular reasons, your doctor will have to weigh the benefits against the risks.

16

Breast Cancer

What You Can Do to Protect Yourself

Breast cancer is less common than cardiovascular disease—and your likelihood of getting it may be less than you think—but it's important to discuss here because your risk does increase as you reach menopause and in the successive years. Breast cancer is the most common form of cancer in women (though not the most common cause of cancer death, which is lung cancer). According to the National Cancer Institute, a woman has about a 1 in 8 (12 percent) chance of being diagnosed with breast cancer at some time during her life, meaning the chance that she'll never have breast cancer is 87.1 percent, or about 7 in 8. The chance of dying from breast cancer is about 1 in 43 (about 2.3 percent). Like many illnesses, the risk of developing breast cancer increases with age. At age thirty, a woman's chance of being diagnosed with breast cancer is 1 in 204; at age fifty, 1 in 42; at age seventy, 1 in 24.

These are numbers for all women of all races combined, but they don't tell the whole story. Black women have a lower risk of getting breast cancer than white women; however, they tend to get breast cancer at a younger age, are diagnosed later in the cancer's progression, and mostly because of that reason are at greater risk of dying from breast cancer than women who are white, Asian, Pacific Islander, or Native American. Hispanic women's rates and severity of cancers fall somewhere in between. It's not clear whether these differences have a genetic component, but we do know that systemic racism in medicine undeniably impacts the quality of care of Black women, including breast cancer care. Black women are not screened for breast cancer as frequently as other women, which means that the cancer is not caught in the more treatable early stages. Black women also tend to experience more chronic stress, and stress, too, can contribute to both the development of cancer and its severity through inflammation.

Wherever you fall on this spectrum of risk, early detection is key. Truthfully, in midlife, there aren't a lot of things you can do to prevent breast cancer, though we'll talk about some healthy habits that may help. What's more important as you're entering menopause and for the rest of your life is staying on top of your breast health so you can prevent advanced cancer. In this chapter, we'll talk about how breast cancer develops and outline the kinds of screening you may need going forward.

Why Risk Increases Now

Breast cancer seems to come out of nowhere. One day you're going about your life as normal, and the next you're getting a call telling you there is something suspicious on your mammogram. But breast cancer actually develops over the course of a woman's lifetime. It takes multiple genetic insults to breast cells before they turn cancerous, a gathering of age-related injuries to the cells and the fundamental DNA inside them that occur as you age. That's why breast cancer risk increases as you get older—it can occur in any woman, but it's more likely to happen in your sixties, seventies, and even eighties, if it does.

Every cell has to repair itself from time to time, and sometimes the repair doesn't go so well. All cancer can be traced back to this kind of cell maintenance gone wrong, where instead of mending correctly, the cell enters into a massive growth pattern. Certain inherited gene differences may make your repair system even more prone to dysfunction, and that can increase your risk of getting certain cancers. For breast cancer, two of these gene differences are mutations on the BRCA1 and BRCA2 genes.

Everyone has the BRCA1 and BRCA2 genes. Usually, these genes work like little mechanics, supplying proteins that repair damaged DNA and keeping the cells in good working order. But genetic mutations can interfere with the genes' ability to provide repair, setting the stage for cancer: Women with the mutations have up to an 87 percent risk of getting breast cancer during their lifetime. While less common, men can get breast cancer, too, and their risk increases with BRCA mutations as well. BRCA mutations also increase the risk of ovarian, pancreatic, and melanoma cancers, although they're rarer—a woman's risk of ovarian cancer, for instance, increases from 1 to 2 percent to 44 percent if she tests positive for the mutation.

Inheriting the gene doesn't mean you'll get cancer for certain, but it does increase the odds exponentially. If you're of Ashkenazi (Eastern or Central European) Jewish descent or have had family members, including male family members, who developed breast and/or ovarian cancer, you also have a higher likelihood of having the BRCA mutation. If someone in your family has tested positive for a BRCA mutation or you suspect you may have a genetic risk, we strongly recommend seeking out a genetic counselor to talk about whether or not you want to get tested yourself.

While your likelihood of being diagnosed with breast cancer is less influenced by lifestyle choices than your likelihood of contracting cardiovascular disease, there are a number of factors that can raise breast cancer risk over the course of your lifetime. Many of them will actually be familiar from the last chapter. The first is smoking. Smoking is bad for your health for a lot of reasons, but there is a direct link to cancer because smoking damages the ability of your cells to repair themselves. And not just your lung cells, but all cells. Smoking puts you at higher risk for all cancers, including breast cancer: If you currently smoke and have been smoking for more than ten years, you may have a 10 percent higher risk of breast cancer than if you had never smoked.

Alcohol consumption has also been associated with breast cancer, and the more you drink, the higher your risk. An analysis of fifty-three studies that included 58,515 women with invasive breast cancer and 95,067 controls found that women who had two to three alcoholic drinks per day had a 20 percent higher risk of breast cancer than women who didn't drink.

Red meat consumption has been linked to higher risks of cancer, at least in the United States (there may be a difference worldwide because meat is produced differently in other countries). Some of the information on meat eating and breast cancer is culled from the Sister Study, an investigation of environmental and genetic risk factors for breast cancer and other diseases among 50,884 sisters of women who have had breast cancer. The study, led by the National Institute of Environmental Health Sciences, found that the women who ate the most red meat compared to those who ate the least red meat had a modestly increased risk of breast cancer. Women who ate the most poultry compared to those who ate the least poultry had a modestly decreased risk of breast cancer. Women who ate seafood had neither an increased nor a decreased risk.

This doesn't necessarily mean that eliminating red meat from your diet will help reduce your risk of breast cancer, though it will help with other things, like cardiovascular health. Breast cancer tends to develop over many years, so by the time you hit midlife, you've probably eaten red meat for a long time, and your body has already had lifelong exposure to whatever it is in meat that may increase risk. In other words, the forty years of meat eating you did earlier has likely already taken its toll.

That said, it's never too late to turn vegan or vegetarian for other health reasons. This is all just information for you to collect as you assess your risk and make decisions accordingly.

Obesity may also impact breast cancer risk, but the relationship between the two is less clear. When looking into the association between body fat and cancer, the International Agency for Research on Cancer Working Group concluded that higher amounts of body fat are associated with an increased risk of thirteen types of cancers, most especially endometrial and esophageal. Breast cancer is farther down on the risk list: People who are obese are 1.2 to 1.4 times as likely to get breast cancer as someone who is not overweight, and the risk increases 1.2 times for every 5-unit increase in body mass index (BMI).

It's also important to note that the studies that show a link between body weight and cancer are observational. There's an association, but no evidence of causality. It may be that many people who are overweight also have other habits that bump up their cancer risks. Still, we know that being obese also comes with conditions like diabetes, which increases blood levels of insulin, and insulin can cause tumor proliferation. People with high levels of body fat also have higher levels of the hormone leptin, which promotes cell growth, including cancer cell growth. But if you're overweight and otherwise healthy, it's not clear that losing weight will impact your risk of breast cancer at all.

Hormones and Breast Cancer

In many women's minds, hormones and breast cancer are inextricably linked, but the relationship is more nuanced than it may seem. Studies have shown that there is a small increase in risk of breast cancer while you're taking birth control pills. The absolute increase in risk is 1 case for every 7,690 women using combined hormone contraception. For young women, who are already at a fairly low risk of the disease, that rate drops to 1 in 50,000. And the risk goes down after you stop taking the pill; five years later it reverts to the same risk as someone who never took the pill. Progesterone-only pills are not linked to breast cancer, and combined hormone pills are linked to a decreased risk of uterine and ovarian cancer, something else to consider.

There is not as much data on other hormone-based types of birth control, but so far Depo-Provera, the birth control ring, and the birth control patch have not been associated with an increased risk of breast cancer. The data on hormone-releasing IUDs is mixed but primarily shows little increase in risk.

The elevation in risk associated with MHT is approximately 1 case per 1,000 women for all women, whether or not you have a family history of cancer. But it's important to highlight that this rise in risk is associative, not causative. Not all types of breast cancer are hormone-sensitive. (Cancers are considered hormone-sensitive if hormones feed the cancer cells' growth.) And even those that are hormone-sensitive are not necessarily *caused* by hormones—the breast tissue has been exposed to hormones for years, so the additional hormones from MHT are not necessarily a factor in the development of cancer. When breast cancer is diagnosed within two to three years of starting menopausal hormone therapy, it probably has been developing for six to nine years before it was discovered, so it may be related to MHT or it may not. Something else to bear in mind is that women on MHT who get breast cancer do not die at a higher rate than women who get the disease but are not on MHT.

None of this is to say that MHT, birth control pills, IUDs, and other forms of hormone-based medications are risk-free. It's still very important to weigh the impact of hormones and to discuss the risks with your physician, especially if you have other breast cancer risk factors. But we want to put those risks in perspective so that they can be appropriately weighed against the benefits—both for health and quality of life—of hormone therapies for many perimenopausal women.

Managing Risk

Unfortunately, unlike cardiovascular disease, there isn't much you can do to lower your risk of breast cancer. Avoiding the things that raise your risk can help a bit, but with breast cancer, what we primarily talk about is screening with mammograms. Early detection can help catch cancer in its early stages when it has a higher likelihood of being treatable. You want to do as much as possible to catch breast cancer before it becomes advanced.

Different medical societies recommend different screening schedules, but the one we endorse (and that is also endorsed by the American College of Obstetricians and Gynecologists and many other societies) is to get a mammogram every one to two years starting at age forty, and yearly starting at age fifty. Other groups may recommend less frequency because they're taking into account cost or more heavily weighting the psychological cost of a false positive, but we feel early detection is more important. That's never been truer than right now, because we're seeing more cancer in forty-year-olds and more aggressive cancers across ages than ever before.

Research shows that routine screening lowers the rate of breast cancer deaths in women forty to seventy-five years old. After seventy-five, there's some controversy about when to stop getting mammograms. In much older patients, the calculation is based on weighing the benefits of early detection against the potential pitfalls of screening. Beyond false positives, we're more likely to see overdiagnosis in older women, in which there is cancer, but it may be so slow growing (or not growing at all) that treating it is unnecessary. The cancers we see in women in their seventies and eighties tend to grow slowly, so they are generally not lethal. Most women who develop breast cancer at this stage will die of something else, and some research shows that even when breast cancer is found in older women, they don't die at higher rates than women who were not screened.

In one study, published in 2023 by Yale Cancer Center and School of Medicine, women aged seventy to seventy-four were followed for almost fourteen years; women aged seventy-five to eighty-four were studied for about ten years; and women aged eighty-five and older for about five and a half years. More cancers were found in the women who were screened, but there was no difference in the number of cancers that were diagnosed at the more-deadly advanced stages or in deaths from breast cancer. This is valuable but not definitive data. The question of a screening stop date hasn't been settled and remains something that's a judgment call between you and your physician.

But if you're forty years old, it's an easy call. Get a mammogram every year going forward, and worry about when to stop later. When you begin at age forty and have a mammogram every year, we can also look to see if there are changes over time. Mammograms reveal less when you are young due to the density of the breasts; however, if you're screened every year, we can pick up change over time, which can lead to earlier diagnosis.

Another question that comes up in regard to screening is whether or not a woman might need additional testing, such as mammograms more than once a year or the inclusion of other techniques such as ultrasound or magnetic resonance imaging (MRI). We can't give additional testing to everyone—we simply don't have the resources—but some women really benefit from extra precautions. There's important ongoing research called the WISDOM (Women Informed to Screen Depending on Measures of Risk) study that's trying to find much more precise determinants for who needs additional screening. Although we typically use family history as a gauge for whether someone needs more intensive screening than an annual mammogram, the WISDOM researchers found that 67 percent of women who get breast cancer have no family history. So family history alone is not actually a great marker for enhanced screening. Instead, WISDOM is looking at whether personalized screening schedules should be based on a combination of factors, including genetic risk, lifestyle, and breast density. And they're looking beyond the BRCA mutations to see if other, tiny gene defects are shared by women who develop breast cancer. Ultimately, we hope that one day we'll have more exact factors for determining risk and, therefore, screening protocols.

In the meantime, should you also get an ultrasound or MRI for breast cancer screening? If you have denser breast tissue, ultrasounds can pick up some breast cancers that mammograms alone do not, but you're likely better off just getting regular mammograms. Even if you have dense breasts, a radiologist can identify cancer based on changes to the tissue over time. Having a mammogram yearly will allow the radiologist to pick up changes, even if the breasts are harder to see through. If there is cause for concern, an MRI is actually a better tool for cancer detection than an ultrasound, but we don't recommend MRI screenings unless you have other risk factors. The current recommendation guidelines are: People with high lifetime risk (20 percent or greater risk in ten years) should have extra screening with MRI and mammograms. Your doctor can calculate your risk using one of several risk models.

Fear of breast cancer can make you want to have every type of screening possible, but MRIs can be expensive, especially if you're not considered at high risk. The type of MRI used for breast cancer screening—a contrast MRI, where dye is injected into you while you lie prone for forty minutes with your breasts in a box—is also an uncomfortable procedure with potential side effects. Mammograms are not perfect, but we have many, many years of experience with them, and we know how to read them. And technology is constantly improving the accuracy of mammogram detection.

REBECCA'S BREAST CANCER EXPERIENCE

During the COVID-19 pandemic, when I was forty-seven years old, I was diagnosed with breast cancer. It's never a good time to get a cancer diagnosis, but the pandemic was an especially bad time. Luckily my cancer was caught early, and all things considered, I came through the ordeal well. I have now been cancer free for five years.

It began, as these things generally do, with alarming test results. I have a genetic difference that puts me at a higher risk for breast cancer plus a strong family history of the disease: Both my paternal aunts and my mother had breast cancer. Added to that was the fact that I had very dense breasts, making it difficult to get a clear view of anything in a mammogram. Because the combination of all these factors made me a candidate for screening beyond the usual yearly mammogram, my primary care doctor wrote to my health insurance company and asked them to cover added testing. They said yes and agreed to pay for screening every six months, alternating between a mammogram and magnetic resonance imaging (MRI).

It was a good thing they did. My very first MRI found lesions in both breasts, six total, that hadn't shown up on the mammogram. Two of the lesions were biopsied, and they both showed cancer—invasive ductal carcinoma—in both breasts. I was then faced with a decision. Did I want to treat the cancer with lumpectomies, or did I want to have a bilateral (double) mastectomy? I chose the bilateral mastectomy. Although we knew that there were multiple lesions in each breast, my doctors had only biopsied two, one on each side. We didn't know if the unbiopsied lesions were cancerous or not. If I was going to have lumpectomies, I was also going to have to go back for more biopsies to figure out if any other lesions had to be removed. I also knew I would continue to need alternating mammograms and MRIs if I had lumpectomies, and likely there would be additional biopsies pretty frequently whenever something was detected. It seemed like a lot to go through and, I decided, not the right approach for me.

And, as it turned out, opting for the mastectomy was the correct choice because my doctors ultimately found three cancers on each side. What they didn't find, thankfully, was any cancer cells in my lymph nodes. The cancer had not spread, so I didn't need any chemotherapy or radiation. But the ordeal wasn't over. Seven months after the mastectomy, I had breast reconstruction surgery and my uterus and ovaries removed.

The removal of my uterus and ovaries was prophylactic. My genetic makeup also put me at risk for ovarian cancer, and the ongoing treatment to prevent a recurrence of breast cancer raised my risk of uterine cancer, too. Because the type of breast cancer I had was hormone-sensitive—that is, it feeds on estrogen—I now take tamoxifen, a drug that prevents estrogen from binding to cells in the breast, thereby lowering the likelihood of the cancer returning. Tamoxifen, though, can increase the risk of precancer or cancer of the uterine lining—but not if you don't have a uterus. Having a hysterectomy was another preventive measure that I chose.

Because of this experience, I have a firsthand understanding of how vitally important regular screening is. Although I had a family history of breast cancer, my family members developed the disease in their late fifties and early sixties. There was no reason to suspect I would get it at age forty-seven. And while I'm fine, it's possible that if the cancer were discovered six months later, that would not be true. Given that mine were the type of tumors that can easily spread (metastasize), catching them early was a literal lifesaver.

There are two other types of screening available that we actually don't recommend: the thermogram, and the breast self-exam. Thermograms are advertised as an alternative to a mammogram. These were briefly taken seriously, but research didn't show that they were effective, so they are "cleared" by the FDA (meaning they're not considered harmful) but are not approved. While a thermogram isn't harmful in the immediate sense, it can be harmful if patients use it as their main detection method since it has a 60 percent false negative rate—meaning that 60 percent of the time when cancer was present, a thermogram didn't catch it. It's a terrible detection tool.

Many of the people who sell thermogram imaging make up scary stories about all the radiation you get from mammograms, and how because mammogram machines squash your breasts, they break open the cancers and spread them throughout your body. None of that is true. The radiation you get from a mammogram is less than you get walking around in the world over the course of two weeks (there are radioactive elements in our atmosphere). The mammogram machine, while far from delightful, does not break open, squash, or otherwise spread cancer.

Breast self-exams used to be very common, so you may be surprised to learn that we no longer recommend this as a tool. So many of us who grew up in the eighties and nineties had those shower cards that told us how to examine our breasts. It was recommended that women do it regularly, but it turned out that the self-exam caused a lot of stress (*Am I doing it right?*) and didn't really pick up that many incidences of cancer. That said, it's still important to be aware of your breasts and to be aware if something changes. If something does change, we recommend going to see a doctor who can assess it and order you a diagnostic (more detailed) mammogram. And it is really important to go in rather than just requesting a mammogram right away—your doctor needs to be able to palpate the lump to determine if it is concerning, and so they can tell the radiologist exactly where it is. That will ensure you get better care if a diagnostic mammogram is genuinely needed.

WHAT OTHER CANCERS SHOULD YOU SCREEN FOR?

Just as early detection of breast cancer is your best hope for successful treatment, so is catching any type of cancer early. There aren't reliable screenings for every type of cancer, but fortunately we do have a few. Here is a guide to the ones you should be thinking about, plus when and how often to have them.

DISEASE	SCREENING	TIMETABLE
Colon cancer	Colonoscopy	Start at age forty-five; repeat every 10 years unless you are advised otherwise by your practitioner.
Cervical cancer	Pap smear and/or HPV test	Start having Pap smears at age twenty-one; repeat every 3 years. From age thirty to sixty-five, you can have both a Pap test and an HPV test every 5 years; a Pap test alone every 3 years; or HPV testing alone every 5 years as long as your results are normal. Abnormal results require more frequent screening and/or additional treatment.
Vulvar cancers	Annual exam	Even if you don't have a Pap smear every year, someone needs to look at your nether regions. This can take place during your yearly gynecological exam.
Ovarian cancer	No reliable test available	We're including this even though there's no good way to screen for it. Barbara Goff, MD, professor and chair of obstetrics and gynecology at the University of Washington School of Medicine in Seattle, has written about the myth of ovarian cancer as a "silent killer." In fact, there are many signs to watch for. If you have pelvic pain, bloating, vaginal bleeding, urinary and/ or gastric symptoms, see your doctor.
Melanoma and other skin cancers	Annual exam	Have your primary care doctor do a skin cancer check during your annual exam. If you have a family history of melanoma, see a dermatologist yearly.

Bone Density

Now Is the Time to Prevent Breaks Later

Not long ago, a patient named Alex came in to see Amy. At forty-seven, Alex was trying to decide if she should go on menopausal hormone therapy to combat her late-perimenopausal symptoms. As Alex and Amy were talking through the risks and benefits of MHT, Alex said, "Oh, by the way, I've had several fractures in the past two years." Amy asked her what kind of fractures. "I fell, and I broke my ankle," said Alex. "Then I fell again, and I broke my other ankle. Then I fell and broke my wrist. So I've had three surgeries in two years to repair fractures."

Alarm bells began ringing in Amy's head—as they had been in Alex's. Women in their forties shouldn't be breaking their wrists. Or their ankles. By her own admission, Alex is kind of clumsy, but she'd never broken a bone before despite other falls. Now, all of a sudden, she had had three successive breaks. She'd asked her doctor for a bone density test (dual-energy X-ray absorptiometry, or DEXA scan) but was told she was too young to need a scan. Amy disagreed, and when Alex's DEXA scan results came back, the cause of her breaks became clear: osteoporosis.

Osteoporosis, a condition that occurs when bones lose density, making them more fragile, is uncommon at Alex's age, but her story does highlight the importance of prioritizing bone health at this stage. New research shows that bone loss accelerates during the span of ages forty-two to forty-seven, just as perimenopause is beginning. In other words, women start to lose bone even before their estrogen levels start to dip due to perimenopause, and, often, even before their periods become irregular.

We build bone throughout our youth. The bone building usually tapers off around age thirty-five; then we go into maintenance mode. But some people are better able to maintain bone density than others. By the time a woman reaches the average age of menopause, fifty-one, she has a 5 to 20 percent risk of developing osteoporosis in the ensuing years (parsed, it breaks down as a 20 percent risk for white and Asian women, 10 percent risk for Latina women, and 5 percent risk for Black women). To put it in perspective, consider that, as reported by the Bone Health & Osteoporosis Foundation, a woman's likelihood of breaking a hip—a common result of osteoporosis—is equal to her combined risk of breast, uterine, and ovarian cancer. And this is one of those diseases that is disproportionately female: 80 percent of the estimated 10 million Americans with osteoporosis are women.

WHEN SHOULD YOU HAVE A BONE DENSITY SCAN?

Just as there are generally accepted recommendations for having mammograms, there are also recommendations that govern most decisions about bone density scans. A duel-energy X-ray absorptiometry (DEXA) scan passes a high- and low-energy X-ray beam through the body, usually in the hip and the spine, to measure bone density. The rule of thumb in the United States is that when a woman turns sixty-five, she should have a DEXA scan even if she has no risk factors. If she has several risk factors (family history, thyroid disease, anorexia, and so on), the scan should be given as early as age fifty. (Several international medical societies recommend screening for fracture risk in all patients, men and women, beginning at age fifty.)

These recommendations make sense. We, for instance, might scan a patient in her forties if she's had several bone fractures, like Amy's patient Alex. Other risk factors we consider include prolonged steroid use, at least two falls in the last year, a parent's hip fracture, a BMI of less than 20 kg/m², current smoking, and alcohol consumption of three or more drinks a day.

We may also use DEXA scans to aid in the decision-making if a patient is considering menopausal hormone therapy during the menopausal transition. Or if someone is considering going off MHT, we might say, "Let's look at your bones first," to see if it may warrant staying on hormones longer. So DEXA scans don't have to be just a routine check. They can help in decision-making and also give you a baseline number so that you can check down the line to see if your bone density changes.

Bones can seem mysterious. We can see our muscles bulk up, and we can see them shrink, but anything happening with the muscles' supporting structure, our skeleton, is invisible. You don't know if your bones are strong or not without medical testing. But there are things you can do to help your bones remain strong, despite the natural progression of bone depletion a woman experiences as she ages.

Why Risk Increases Now

Breaking a bone is never fun, but when you're young, recovery is usually relatively easy. This isn't always true when you're older. That's when a bone break can be deadly. Older adults have a five- to eight-times higher risk of dying within the first three months of a hip fracture. When someone elderly is incapacitated by a break (and it might even be something other than a hip, such as a vertebral bone in the spine), they stop moving around, they stop exercising, and they stop socializing with others, all of which put them at higher cardiovascular risk. Death comes not from a broken bone but usually from something like a heart attack or stroke. If the break requires surgery, it's also possible to die of a postsurgical infection. It's just really hard to recover from a broken hip when you're in your senior years. And even if you do recover, you may not be able to live independently because, during the time you're laid up, you lose so much muscle mass that it's difficult to build back up enough to care for yourself.

When you're in your thirties, forties, or even early fifties, this scenario can feel very faraway and abstract. But your body is now setting the stage for what lies ahead. And the numbers are alarming: Four out of five cases of osteoporosis in the United States are in women, and women over sixty have twice the risk of fracture as men the same age. Women's bones are smaller and thinner than men's to begin with, which is one reason they're more vulnerable to fractures. Another reason is that hormones (primarily estrogen for women, testosterone for men) are intimately connected to bone strength. Since estrogen in women—but not testosterone in men—drops steeply with age (testosterone drops, too, but not precipitously), women's bones suffer in tandem. Plus, men and women lose bone in different ways. If you looked at the bones of older people through a high-powered microscope, you'd see that a man's bone has become thinner. A woman's bone, on the other hand, will have developed perforations. Those tiny holes not only weaken the structure more than thinning does, but they also mean that the bone can't be substantially rebuilt.

Although seemingly static, bone tissue is continually active: breaking down and rebuilding itself over the course of your lifetime. This process, called remodeling, helps repair bone tissue damage. Cells known as osteoclasts break down the existing bone tissue, and osteoblast cells rebuild it by depositing calcium and other minerals to keep the bones strong. This continual turnover remains constant and mostly consistent until between the ages of about thirty-five and forty, when the actions of the osteoclasts (bone demolishers) begin to outweigh the actions of the osteoblasts (bone builders). Certain factors can make this imbalance worse, even when you're young. If, for instance, your diet is very low in calcium, there won't be enough of the mineral to support bone rebuilding. People with severe eating disorders are at a particularly high risk for bone loss because a certain blood level of calcium must be maintained to keep the heart beating, and if the body doesn't get any calcium from food, it will start to leach it from the bones.

Some medications and conditions can also impact your bone health. Osteoporosis runs in families, so if one of your parents has it, you may be more prone to develop it as well. Some medications, such as antidepressants and diabetes drugs, can weaken bones. Oral steroids used to combat autoimmune diseases can cause the body's bone breakdown actions to exceed its bone-building measures. Thyroid disorders can pose a risk to the bones, too. The thyroid gland helps regulate many systems in the body, and the rate of bone turnover is among them. If you have an overactive thyroid (hyperthyroidism), it can speed up the pace of bone breakdown to a point where bone rebuilding can't keep up. Medication to improve thyroid function will help, but if you went a long time undiagnosed, some bone deterioration may have already happened. If you suffer from the opposite condition, an underactive thyroid (hypothyroidism), that won't affect bone per se. However, if the dose of medication used to correct it is too high, it can impact bone density. Diseases like rheumatoid arthritis, Crohn's disease, and inflammatory bowel syndrome can increase your risk as well. If you have a thyroid condition or any of these risk factors, your bone density may need to be monitored earlier than the standard recommended age of sixty-five.

For most women without a thyroid condition or other extenuating circumstances, bone composition mostly holds steady; then bone loss picks up once you reach the perimenopausal years. One factor, especially in late perimenopause, is the overall reduction in estrogen levels. Even though estrogen levels are yo-yoing during perimenopause, they're also beginning to recede, and that affects the remodeling process. Estrogen nudges the cells that make new bone tissue; with less estrogen in the body, bone-building osteoblasts are less active.

Newer research suggests that in the earlier part of perimenopause, follicle stimulating hormone (FSH) may be a large contributing factor to the slow decline in bone health. Hormones generally have more than one job, and another of FSH's tasks is to promote the breakdown of bone tissue. Usually, this effect is mitigated by estrogen, but in perimenopause, the ovaries are less responsive to FSH, causing the brain to produce extra FSH in order to get the expected response. Having additional FSH in the system may cause bone tissue destruction to outpace bone tissue reconstruction and contribute to the acceleration of bone loss that characterizes the menopausal transition.

Reducing Risk

Some of the lifestyle elements that raise your risk of other diseases, like smoking and drinking, can also make you more vulnerable to bone loss. It might come as a surprise, but smoking almost doubles the risk of hip fracture. In a review of studies published in *Osteoporosis International*, researchers looked at the effects of alcohol on bone, and concluded that four or more drinks per day can be harmful, interfering with remodeling and making it more difficult to absorb nutrients that shore up the skeleton. Given alcohol's effects on cardiovascular health and cancer risk as well, it's likely that the less you drink, the better.

Likewise, some of the things you can do to help strengthen your bones and mitigate bone loss are similar to our recommendations for cardiovascular health and lowering cancer risk. Nutrition plays an outsize role in bone density, and as we've mentioned many times, strength training is one of the best things you can do not just for your muscles but for your bones as well.

Eating for Bone Health

What you eat has a direct relationship with your bone health. The minerals calcium and phosphorus provide the building blocks for bone; other minerals, like magnesium, assist in the bone remodeling process. Protein is important, too, since some of the bone is made up of collagen, a type of protein. These are all nutrients you need to eat; your body won't make them, so if you're not getting enough of them in your diet, it will increase your osteoporosis risk.

Calcium, as many people are aware, is the most important mineral where bones are concerned. If you're under fifty, you need 1,000 mg a day; if you're over fifty, the recommended daily dose rises to 1,200 mg. Dairy products like milk and yogurt are the sources richest in calcium, but not the only sources: green vegetables like collards, kale, broccoli, and bok choy contain ample amounts of the mineral, too. Many foods, such as juices and plant-based milks, are also fortified with calcium. Tofu, when it's prepared with calcium sulfate, which it usually is, is calcium-rich as well.

The body absorbs calcium from food better than it does calcium from a supplement; plus the calcium in food comes along with other nutrients that also help with bone protection and overall good health. But if you're not meeting the recommendation, it's worthwhile to take a calcium supplement. (Calcium calculators, available online, can help you determine your average intake.) Just don't go overboard with supplementation; more is not better. Going too far over the recommendation can lead to kidney stones and even contribute to the development of plaque in your arteries.

Vitamin D is also vitally important, as it facilitates the absorption of calcium from food and helps regulate the bone-building process. The good news is that our bodies can create vitamin D through exposure to sunlight every couple of days. The bad news is that the amount of sunlight you need can be variable. People with lighter skin may need only eight to ten minutes of exposure if a lot of skin is exposed due to summer clothes. But if you have darker skin, you may need more time, and everybody may need more in the winter, when our skin is more covered. Geography plays a part, too. If you live somewhere like Seattle, it's difficult to get enough sunlight to prompt the production of vitamin D. Even in sunnier climes, if you're wearing sunscreen (and you should be), it can interfere with vitamin D production. Be aware, too, that as you age, your body will make less vitamin D, even with proper sun exposure.

It's possible to get some vitamin D through food. Fatty fish like tuna, trout, and salmon contain vitamin D, as do egg yolks and mushrooms (as long as they were grown outdoors in the sun). Mushrooms also contain calcium, which makes them an all-around good bone food. If you're not getting enough vitamin D (your doctor can order a D test as part of your blood panel when you go for a checkup), you may benefit from a supplement—from both a bone and a perimenopause perspective. Our perimenopausal patients often complain of fatigue, and a vitamin D deficiency can sometimes be related to low energy. Here again, you don't want to over-supplement; you just want to get into the normal range of vitamin D. We usually recommend supplementing with 1,000 to 2,000 IU a day, unless your levels are severely low.

Although it's important to pay attention to these individual nutrients, the overall nutritional quality of your diet is also key. Some research, for instance, shows that eating a Mediterranean diet can protect against osteoporosis. There's evidence, too, that the more fruit- and vegetable-rich your diet, the better for your bones. On the other hand, a typical Western diet, full of cheese, processed meat, pastries, pizza, French fries, and refined grains, is associated with low bone density.

And a diet high in salt can cause the body to excrete calcium, lowering the amount available for bone rebuilding.

While you may be tempted to diet in response to midlife weight gain, we have to reiterate that it's better to ensure that the food on your plate is healthy than it is to restrict your caloric intake. Being a very restrictive eater and/or being underweight can take a toll on bones—the people most at risk for osteoporosis are skinny white women. While you may not be thrilled by the shifts in your body weight and composition during this time, there are positives to the weight women typically put on during perimenopause and menopause. One benefit is that belly fat produces some estrogen, and that estrogen will improve the bone remodeling cycle. Plus, part of the reason that bones break down and rebuild is to adapt to stress. Weight puts "good stress" on the bones, helping them build back stronger. If you're very thin and lack those stress-inducing pounds, your bones won't get the message to build back stronger.

Exercise

Physical activity—specifically weightlifting and/or other weight-bearing activities—similarly puts good stress on bones and so is critical to bone health. A sedentary life, in fact, is a big risk factor for osteoporosis. Weight-bearing exercise refers to activity that requires supporting yourself with your legs and feet as you move. The movement adds extra force that stresses the bones. Weight-bearing activity can be as simple as brisk walking, or if you can step it up, running, hiking, dancing and dance-type exercise classes, jumping rope, stair-climbing, racquet sports, and court sports like basketball, soccer, and volleyball. The higher the impact of the activity and the more rapidly it's performed, the more adaptive activity it will trigger in the bones. Weight-bearing exercise largely benefits the lower part of the skeleton, the legs and hips, unless you add a weighted vest or backpack to increase the burden on the upper body (which we recommend—it's a great way to make your walks more robust while having a healthy impact on your spine and torso).

We recommend pairing weight-bearing exercises with weight training. Mixing in weight training will also allow you to challenge the bones in the upper body, including your arms. As you lift weights, your muscles tug on the bones, prompting that rebuilding response that keeps them sturdy. You actually cause a little bit of trauma, and that prompts remodeling. While weight lifting can be enormously beneficial for perimenopausal women, moderate lifting or strength training with resistance bands is sufficient for getting the bone-building benefits. Pilates and yoga have not been found to substantially increase bone density, but these disciplines—along with the aforementioned types of exercise—can all contribute to helping you maintain overall fitness and balance, which will lower your risk of falling, a good thing whether or not you have brittle bones.

Medication

Alex, Amy's patient who had three successive bone breaks, ended up going on menopausal hormone therapy, aiming to both reduce her perimenopausal symptoms and improve bone density. Amy also referred her to a bone specialist to discuss more in-depth therapy. MHT is approved by the FDA for prevention of osteoporosis in the United States, and there's good evidence that it works to stem bone loss—it's actually approved to treat osteoporosis in other countries. MHT acts as a kind of dam, holding back the natural deterioration of bone that occurs with age and estrogen loss. However, it only works as long as you take it—once you stop taking it, bone density declines. In a few years, it's back where it would have been if you'd never taken MHT at all. That's why many women, especially those who may have low bone mass (formally known as osteopenia) or a concerning family history of bone loss, barring any other potential risks, stay on MHT for longer than perimenopausal/menopausal symptoms would generally warrant.

If you have a bone scan and the results are worrisome, your physician can treat you or send you to a specialist. There's a class of drugs called antiresorptive agents that work by interfering with the work of the osteoclasts so that less bone is broken down in the remodeling process. One of these drugs is called bisphosphonates, and they're a great first step for treating low bone density. Your general practitioner or gynecologist can prescribe the pill versions of bisphosphonates, but you may have to go to an endocrinologist to get one of the newer IV-infusion treatments or discuss a treatment plan moving forward.

Because our bones aren't visible, you may not have considered bone health before now, but it's an essential factor in staying healthy and active over the coming decades. While your bones may no longer be building themselves after age thirty-five or so, there's still a lot you can do to strengthen them now and ensure they stay strong for years to come.

Coda

Talking to Your Doctor, Being Heard, and
Taking Control of Your Well-Being

———

A patient named Hailey came into Rebecca's office. They spent twenty minutes together, and during that brief time, Hailey had two hot flashes. "I don't know if you can do anything for me," she said, sweating, her face flushed. "I've been to my primary care doctor, and he said, 'Oh, it's just this phase of life; you have to get through it.' And I went to the guy who delivered my babies, and he said, 'Oh, you know we don't use hormones anymore. You're just going to have to tough it out.'" Hailey had also been to a "longevity clinic," and they offered her testosterone pellets. She didn't have the money to pay for them at the time so (thankfully) she passed.

"This has been going on for ten years," Hailey continued. "For ten years I've been trying to find a doctor who can help me with these hot flashes and other symptoms. I have fifteen a day. I haven't had sex in two years because it's so painful. And I know you're going to tell me you can't help me." Rebecca stopped her right there. "No," she said. "We're going to make you feel better. Today." Hailey was a little further from the menopausal transition than we'd usually recommend for starting menopausal therapy, but Rebecca assessed her cardiovascular risk—all clear—and prescribed estrogen. Three weeks later Hailey came back into the office with a huge bouquet of flowers, hugged every single person at the front desk, and told them that she hadn't felt this good in ten or fifteen years.

The collective way of thinking about the menopausal transition matters deeply to an individual's experience of perimenopause. If, for instance, you're lucky enough to live in a supportive, multigenerational female community with mothers, grandmothers, aunts, and cousins nearby to help you understand and manage symptoms, you may have an easier time with this transition. But one is never assured of empathy and information, and lack of understanding among those you depend on—including those you depend on at work, like colleagues and bosses, as well as the medical community—can be crippling. If your symptoms are dismissed, you're not going to get the help you need in dealing with them. And if there's a communal belief that perimenopause symptoms are shameful, you'll likely feel that they are, too.

As physicians and as women who have been through this transition, we encourage you to remember that all perimenopausal and menopausal experiences are valid. If necessary, look beyond your immediate circle and seek out other women and knowledgeable practitioners who get what you're talking about. We're not miracle workers. We pride ourselves on being very good physicians, but what Rebecca did for Hailey is what every doctor should have done for Hailey and what every doctor should do for you: listen, take you seriously, and look for solutions. Not every problem is solvable—again, doctors are not miracle workers. But you deserve their best efforts.

By the time perimenopausal patients come to see us, they've usually seen several different physicians or other advanced practitioners. They often feel dejected and rejected, dismissed and unheard. Most likely this isn't their healthcare providers' intention. If you don't know much about it—and many practitioners do not—perimenopause can be puzzling, and that leads to poor care. But there's no reason for that to occur, and certainly no reason for someone to wait ten years for relief. In this chapter, we'll outline our four-point recommendation to help you find the right practitioner and get the attention you deserve. If you already love your doctor but know you might need more support, this chapter will still be useful because we can flag the information your doctor needs to know in order to treat you properly. The better you're able to communicate what you're going through, the better the outcome of your visit will likely be.

1. **Find a qualified provider who loves perimenopause.** Believe it or not, some of us do! You may be devoted to the ob-gyn who delivered your children or have complete confidence in your primary care physician, but it's possible that the menopausal transition isn't really their jam. And that's okay. You're transitioning into a new phase, and your usual doctor might not be the best person to captain the ship. This is no fault of your physician. Obstetrics and gynecology and women's health are large, in-depth areas of medicine. Some of us love pregnancy and delivering babies. Others are fascinated by the over-forty population. Some doctors love all of it.

The best way to find out if your current practitioner has specific experience with perimenopause is simply to ask. Your ob-gyn is a good place to start, but your primary care doctor can also be a great resource. More and more primary care physicians are focusing on the menopausal transition. Whomever you ask, be direct: "I need a physician who is well versed in perimenopause. Is this part of your practice?" If they say yes, that's great. If they say no—or if they say yes, but you ultimately find you're not getting what you need—it's okay to look for a different practitioner. It needs to feel like the right fit for both of you.

To find someone new, you have a few options. You can ask your other doctor(s) for a recommendation. If you have a female doctor who is close to your age, you might ask who she sees. You can ask friends and family who they like—word of mouth can be very reliable. Another option is to look on the Menopause Society website (menopause.org), which has a list of physicians and other providers who have an interest in perimenopause and menopause. If they're listed as a Menopause Society Certified Practitioner (MSCP), it means they've taken an exam on menopausal medicine and maintain their credentialing with continuing education. But you don't need to be certified to specialize in this area; Many knowledgeable physicians and other practitioners are not certified.

You can also check your health insurer's portal for providers who list perimenopause/menopause as a specialty. If you're in a geographical area where healthcare professionals are scarce, telehealth may be an option. (Full disclosure: Rebecca is the chief medical officer for Gennev, a telehealth company dedicated to perimenopause and menopausal medicine.) HMOs and academic health centers are another good place to look for doctors who concentrate on the menopausal transition.

You don't have to limit yourself to doctors during this time—nurse practitioners (NPs) can also be a great resource for perimenopausal care. NPs can do a very good job helping perimenopausal patients, and there are many on the Menopause Society website who've taken and passed the certification exam. The difference is that NPs have less organized medical training than physicians and are usually not as well-versed in diagnostics because of this. (Doctors usually have to complete ten years of training, while NP programs are typically two to three years.) That said, an experienced NP who has been seeing perimenopausal patients for years may be perfectly able to identify your needs and provide the right treatment plan. Approach NPs the same way you would a physician—if they meet your needs, that's great. If not, it's okay to look for someone else.

A practitioner will be a good fit for you if you feel comfortable with them, and they listen to you and respond to your needs. You'll generally know if someone's not the right fit, but we also want to highlight a few red flags to look out for:

> ➤ Promotes the use of compounding or "bioidentical" products.
> ➤ Insists on a lot of lab work, including tests you'll have to pay for out of pocket.
> ➤ Uses pellet therapy (and we really mean this one—pass).
> ➤ Sells supplements for profit.
> ➤ Is at a medi-spa. Perimenopause requires care from an official medical office.

2. **Make a perimenopause-specific appointment.** Your annual visit to your gynecologist or the checkup with your primary care doctor is not the best time to get help with your sleep and mood issues, vaginal dryness, night sweats, and other perimenopausal symptoms. A lot of patients tell us that they went to their doctor and were told that the doctor didn't have time to talk about their symptoms; they'd have to come back. We know this can be frustrating, but unfortunately, we have to do this as doctors because of the way insurance is set up: an annual ob-gyn visit, in insurance terms, is a ten-minute visit, where you get a Pap smear and a breast exam, and your doctor makes sure you're up to date on tests like mammograms and colon cancer screenings. You might discuss birth control, too. But there is zero time left over for much of anything else.

If you try to add a discussion of perimenopause on top of the standard items covered by an annual visit, your physician is legally required to code that visit for insurance as an annual wellness checkup plus "problem" visit, which may raise your co-pay. More importantly, it means you'll be shortchanged on time because the visit is set up to account for just the usual well visit items. Talking about perimenopause takes time. Don't cheat yourself out of a proper back-and-forth dialogue with your provider. When you make the appointment, be clear about what you're coming in for. That's the best way to ensure that there will be time to really focus on your symptoms, and your questions, and to talk through a perimenopausal management strategy.

3. **Be patient.** Perimenopause doesn't start in a day, and it can rarely be fully solved in a day either. It can take multiple visits to get a handle on symptoms, and just when you think you've got everything under control, a new symptom might pop up or intensify. Maybe hot flashes aren't an issue now, but they may develop as you get closer to your final menstrual period and require a new approach to treatment. So it's important to be patient and know that finding the right treatment may take time. Your physician will generally have a methodology for going forward, and you should feel free to ask about this if you're feeling frustrated. We often start by addressing the top symptoms on a patient's list in the first visit, then make adjustments and tackle other concerns over the course of subsequent follow-up appointments. It often takes a few visits before we have a fully functioning plan. And some symptoms are particularly challenging. Lack of libido is one example of a symptom that often needs its own stand-alone appointment because it's complicated and multifactorial and can require its own dedicated treatment plan.

Perimenopause can last a decade before you hit menopause, which is why it's so important to find a practitioner you like and can have a lasting relationship with. You and your doctor will likely need to adjust and pivot as your body throws new and interesting curveballs. Don't give up—and don't give up on your practitioner if you don't get it right with the initial treatment plan, as long as they're listening to you and they clearly explain their recommendations. Medicine, as we've noted earlier in this book, is as much art as science. Each person is so unique. Your doctor will want to find the approach that's just right for you, and that may take some time.

4. **Come prepared.** While your doctor will have some sense of the best questions to ask, you can improve the likelihood that all your perimenopausal issues get tackled if you come to your appointment armed with the relevant information. We've outlined some of the key information we recommend bringing to your doctor below. It can also be helpful to develop a clear sense of what kinds of symptoms might appear, even if you're not experiencing them now, as well as the treatments available. (That's why we wrote this book!)

We do, however, want to make a point of noting that not all sources of information are created equal. If you're reading this, you're probably the kind of person who has looked up your symptoms online or seen information about perimenopause on social media and wants a better sense of what to expect. While we think everyone should do some of their own research so they know what to ask and what to expect, we also want to highlight that a lot of information online may be anecdotal or even entirely false. The best thing to do is to be aware of where the information you're getting is coming from—the discussion of understanding research studies on page 255 can help you here—then ask your doctor if you have questions about what you've found. The best course of action is to establish a trusting, mutually respectful relationship with your clinician so you can figure out the best plan of action together.

THE PERIMENOPAUSE APPOINTMENT CHECKLIST

PERIODS AND BIRTH CONTROL

- Do you have periods? If no, why not? (E.g., they've stopped, you had a hysterectomy, you have an IUD, and so on.)

- If you're having periods, how often do you have them (first day to first day), are they regular or irregular, has the interval between periods become longer or shorter than before, and are they heavier or lighter than you've been used to?

- Can you become pregnant? Do you have a fertile partner? Have you had any procedures (like a sterilization) that might prohibit pregnancy?

- Would you want to become pregnant? If no, how are you currently preventing it?

MEDICATIONS AND HEALTH ISSUES

- Make sure to have a current list of your medical diagnoses, allergies, and medications with you when you go to your appointment.

- Especially important to mention:
    - Migraines, and if you have them, whether you have them with aura. Also, how do they change with menstruation?
    - Any blood clots in your history and when they occurred.
    - Any cardiovascular disease (such as a history of heart disease, heart surgery, or stroke).
    - Any cancer history.
    - History of a meningioma (brain tumor).

➤ History of hemangioma (noncancerous tumors) in your liver.

➤ History of a condition (like hyperthyroidism) or medication (such as steroids) use that could impact your bone health.

➤ History of bone fractures.

➤ History of anxiety or depression.

➤ History of sleep disturbances or sleep apnea.

FAMILY HEALTH HISTORY

- First-degree relative with breast or ovarian cancer.

- Family history of uterine and colon cancers.

- Family history of cardiovascular disease.

- Family history of blood clotting disorders.

- Family history of osteoporosis or bone fractures.

CURRENT SYMPTOMS

- Make a list of everything you're experiencing, even if it might not be related. Also, make sure to note which of these are having the biggest impact on your quality of life. Be candid, and don't leave out important things like vaginal symptoms or sex drive.

- What treatments have you already tried to make things better? This can be anything from lifestyle changes to herbs, supplements, and medications.

GOALS

- What do you want to get out of your visit? ("Being heard," "Solutions," "Education," "Is this perimenopause?" "WTF!" are all good answers here.)

We know that doctors can be intimidating, but remember that they're just people, like you, and most of them went into the profession to assist others—they *want* to help you feel better. The Perimenopause Appointment Checklist is a great place to start if you're not sure what to bring up, but overall you should feel free to speak your mind and ask for what you need. Remember that you're not being difficult or demanding by simply telling your story, giving the details about what you're going through, and expecting a good outcome. Your doctor is there to help.

The most important takeaway we hope you get from this book is validation that the symptoms you're experiencing are real, they can be a real pain, and also, you *will* get through them. Even if perimenopause is underdiscussed, it is widely experienced, and there are so many ways to make it easier and more bearable. Your quality of life matters! We hope this book can serve as a guide for getting through it as smoothly and painlessly as possible.

Acknowledgments

We would like to thank Daryn Eller for her invaluable assistance in putting our voices down on paper. Thanks, too, to editors Julie Will and Hallie Schaeffer and their team for their guidance, and to our agent, Bonnie Solow, for making this project go from musings to published book. We would also like to thank our families for putting up with us talking about perimenopause all the time. Rebecca would like to thank Dr. Steiner and Dr. Honeybrink, who introduced her to evidence-based menopause care early in her career. Amy would like to thank Dr. Paul Blumenthal for his long-standing mentorship and encouragement to find her own path in medicine. Amy would also like to thank her girlfriends—all of whom are on this perimenopausal journey and have made it a time filled with love, support, and laughter.

References

Understanding Research
Studies Like a Data Geek

Before we jump into the reference section, we wanted to share a little bit about how we recommend approaching medical reports and studies, especially when you see a sensational headline splashed across your screen. Medical science nowadays is very complicated. If you're not well trained in the discipline, understanding research studies is hard, particularly because many media-outlet writers tend to look at a summary of a study (the "abstract"), read the conclusion, and run with it when, in fact, the conclusion may not mean much or even be interpreted correctly. You've read about many studies in this book, but they've been vetted by us; you don't have to get into the weeds, because we did it for you. Sometimes the popular press does the same—but not always, and regardless, you can't get the whole story from one headline. So it can be helpful if you know how to read about research with a critical eye. Here are a few questions to ask as you read the medical science headlines.

<u>Who benefits?</u> Good science asks a question with no hope of a particular answer. So when thinking about the value of a study, you always have to start by asking about any potential bias involved. Who's asking the question, and what are they looking for? Are they looking for an

answer, or are they looking for a tool to promote a product they've developed? It doesn't necessarily mean that studies sponsored by pharmaceutical or other types of companies are bad studies. But this is always a question to keep in the back of your mind.

<u>Are checks in place?</u> Rebecca is a clinical researcher. She does studies for drug companies. Drug companies farm studies out to research centers like the one she does work for and that have no skin in the game. Additional guardrails are set forth by the FDA, which builds in a lot of restrictions designed to prevent bias from skewing study results.

Big pharma, as much as it's maligned—and it's far from perfect—has an important role in society. Pharma makes drugs; drugs can save lives. Pharma has to study those drugs to get them to market. As we evaluate those studies, though, we should always ask whether the checks were in place. If you read through a published study—and plenty of them are online—the authors will note the protocols used to guide their research.

<u>What type of study is it?</u> Reading study details may be a little more into the weeds than you want to get, so here's something else you can look for in the description of a study. Is it a randomized controlled trial? These types of studies go a long way toward preventing bias because the subjects in the study are randomly put into groups. For instance, in a study looking at the effects of a pill for, say, freckle removal, some people may receive the pill, while others may get a placebo. Sometimes there will also be a control group that gets nothing at all. It's even better when a study is also what's called double-blind. Double-blind studies use a protocol requiring that the subjects not know what they're getting, and that the investigators be in the dark as well. That's another way of minimizing partiality. Observational studies are another type of research, where groups of people are monitored to look for outcomes.

They may be given a medication or an exposure and observed for a period of time. These can be helpful studies, and a lot of our medical knowledge comes from this type of research, but they are more prone to bias than randomized controlled trials.

<u>What was the study's size?</u> Small studies can have value. They can, for instance, set the stage for future research. But before getting a conclusive answer to a scientific question, there need to be enough people enrolled in a study to validate the results. To find that number, researchers use something called a power calculation, or as it's sometimes called, a sample-size calculation. This calculation basically weaves in the fact that there's a certain amount of change that may happen just by chance, and it comes up with a number that will allow researchers to detect an actual effect of whatever it is they're investigating. In short, how many people do you need to find that effect? This is not something you're going to determine just by reading about a study in a newspaper, but many articles will tell you the size of the study, and this gives you some idea of why, as physicians who often make treatment decisions based on research, we pay greater attention to large studies.

<u>Who was studied?</u> A lot of research is done on white people (especially white men), and people in the middle- and upper-class echelons. That tells us something about white people (especially white men), and people in the middle- and upper-class echelons, but what does it tell us about other races, genders, and economic classes? Does research done in Sweden translate to people living in South Africa? Research doesn't necessarily transcend genetic and cultural differences, and socioeconomic status can have a huge impact on health. This is just another element to bear in mind when you read about studies in the news.

<u>Was it published in a peer-reviewed journal?</u> "Peer-reviewed" means that a study has been vetted by other experts in the field. When

research is published in a peer-reviewed journal, it's more likely to be truthful and valid. It's not an infallible system, but publishing in a peer-reviewed journal enhances a study's integrity.

CHAPTER 1

Amiri, Mina, Maryam Rahmati, Faegheh Firouzi, Fereidoun Azizi, and Fahimeh Ramezani Tehran. "A Prospective Study on the Relationship Between Polycystic Ovary Syndrome and Age at Natural Menopause." *Menopause* 31, no. 2 (2024): 130–37. https://doi.org/10.1097/GME.0000000000002213.

Ellis, Samuel, Daniel W. Franks, Mia Lybkær Kronborg Nielsen, Michael N. Weiss, and Darren P. Croft. "The Evolution of Menopause in Toothed Whales." *Nature* 627, no. 8004 (2024): 579–85. https://doi.org/10.1038/s41586-024-07159-9.

Matevossian, Karine, and Olivia Carpinello. "Polycystic Ovary Syndrome: Menopause and Malignancy." *Clinical Obstetrics and Gynecology* 64, no. 1 (2021): 102–9. https://doi.org/10.1097/GRF.0000000000000560.

Taylor, Kyla W., Kate Hoffman, Kristina A. Thayer, and Julie L. Daniels. "Polyfluoroalkyl Chemicals and Menopause Among Women 20–65 Years of Age (NHANES)." *Environmental Health Perspectives* 122, no. 2 (2014): 145–50. https://doi.org/10.1289/ehp.1306707.

United States Congress. House. Menopause Research and Equity Act of 2023. 118th Congress, 1st session. H.R. 6749. December 13, 2023. https://www.congress.gov/bill/118th-congress/house-bill/6749/text.

CHAPTER 4

Andersen, M. L., L. R. A. Bittencourt, I. B. Antunes, and S. Tufik. "Effects of Progesterone on Sleep: A Possible Pharmacological Treatment for Sleep-Breathing Disorders?" *Current Medicinal Chemistry* 13, no. 29 (2006): 3575–82. https://doi.org/10.2174/092986706779026200.

Harvard Health Publishing Staff. "Common Anticholinergic Drugs Like Benadryl Linked to Increased Dementia Risk." Harvard Health Publishing. Last updated January 9, 2025. https://www.health.harvard.edu/blog/common-anticholinergic-drugs-like-benadryl-linked-to-increased-dementia-risk-20150128812.

Jehan, Shazia, et al. "Obstructive Sleep Apnea: Women's Perspective." *Journal of Sleep Medicine and Disorders* 3, no. 6 (2016): 1064.

Kräuchi, Kurt, Elisa Fattori, Alessandra Giordano, Maria Falbo, Antonella Iadarola, Francesca Aglì, Antonella Tribolo, Roberto Mutani, and Alessandro

Cicolin. "Sleep on a High Heat Capacity Mattress Increases Conductive Body Heat Loss and Slow Wave Sleep." *Physiology & Behavior* 185 (2018): 23–30. https://doi.org/10.1016/j.physbeh.2017.12.014.

Kravitz, Howard M., and Hadine Joffe. "Sleep During the Perimenopause: A SWAN Story." *Obstetrics and Gynecology Clinics of North America* 38, no. 3 (2011): 567–86. https://doi.org/10.1016/j.ogc.2011.06.002.

Lee, Jinju, Youngsin Han, Hyun Hee Cho, and Mee-ran Kim. "Sleep Disorders and Menopause." *Journal of Menopausal Medicine* 25, no. 2 (2019): 83.

Madaeva, Irina, Natalya Semenova, Radzhana M. Zhambalova, Lyubov I. Kolesnikova, and Sergey I. Kolesnikov. "Polysomnographic Pattern of Melatonin Therapy in Perimenopausal Women." *International Journal of Biomedicine* 10, no. 2 (2020): 161–64. https://doi.org/10.21103 /Article10(2)_OA15.

McCurry, Susan M., Katherine A. Guthrie, Charles M. Morin, Nancy F. Woods, Carol A. Landis, Kristine E. Ensrud, Joseph C. Larson, et al. "Telephone-Based Cognitive Behavioral Therapy for Insomnia in Perimenopausal and Postmenopausal Women with Vasomotor Symptoms: A MsFLASH Randomized Clinical Trial." *JAMA Internal Medicine* 176, no. 7 (2016): 913–20. https://doi.org/10.1001/jamainternmed.2016.1795.

Michaud, Julie M., Caitlin T. Waring, Fernanda Medeiros Contini, Meredith E. Burns, John C. Price, Janessa Quintana, Holly A. Concepcion, Hannah V. Deane, and Joseph A. Seggio. "Estradiol Regulates Circadian Responses to Acute and Constant Light Exposure in Female Mice." *Journal of Biological Rhythms* 38, no. 4 (2023): 407–15. https://doi.org/10.1177 /07487304231172069.

Mirer, Anna G., Terry Young, Mari Palta, Ruth M. Benca, Amanda Rasmuson, and Paul E. Peppard. "Sleep-Disordered Breathing and the Menopausal Transition Among Participants in the Sleep in Midlife Women Study." *Menopause* 24, no. 2 (2017): 157–62. https://doi.org/10.1097/GME .0000000000000744.

Pacheco, Danielle. "Best Temperature for Sleep." Sleep Foundation. Accessed July 11, 2025. https://www.sleepfoundation.org/bedroom-environment /best-temperature-for-sleep#references-79195.

CHAPTER 5

Brody, Debra J., and Qiuping Gu. "Antidepressant Use Among Adults: United States, 2015–2018." *NCHS Data Brief*, no. 377 (2020): 1–8.

Cohen, Lee S., Claudio N. Soares, Allison F. Vitonis, Michael W. Otto, and Bernard L. Harlow. "Risk for New Onset of Depression During the Menopausal Transition: The Harvard Study of Moods and Cycles." *Archives of General Psychiatry* 63, no. 4 (2006): 385–90. https://doi.org/10.1001/archpsyc.63.4.385.

Freeman, Ellen W., Mary D. Sammel, David W. Boorman, and Rongmei Zhang. "Longitudinal Pattern of Depressive Symptoms Around Natural Menopause." *JAMA Psychiatry* 71, no. 1 (2014): 36–43. https://doi.org/10.1001/jamapsychiatry.2013.2819.

Hampson, Laura. "New Research Shows Link Between Menopause and Divorce." *Independent*, October 18, 2022. https://www.the-independent.com/life-style/women/menopause-divorce-link-study-b2204312.html.

Huang, Suna, Zhonghai Wang, Danyi Zheng, and Lizhu Liu. "Anxiety Disorder in Menopausal Women and the Intervention Efficacy of Mindfulness-Based Stress Reduction." *American Journal of Translational Research* 15, no. 3 (2023): 2016–24.

Jayson, Sharon. "Divorce Skyrocketing Among Aging Boomers." AARP. Last updated September 6, 2023. https://www.aarp.org/family-relationships/gray-divorce-trend/#:~:text=A%20new%20analysis%20of%20divorce,tripled%20from%201990%20to%202021.

Nakanishi, Miharu, Kaori Endo, Syudo Yamasaki, Daniel Stanyon, Sarah Sullivan, Satoshi Yamaguchi, Shuntaro Ando, et al. "Association Between Menopause and Suicidal Ideation in Mothers of Adolescents: A Longitudinal Study Using Data from a Population-Based Cohort." *Journal of Affective Disorders* 340 (2023): 529–34. https://doi.org/10.1016/j.jad.2023.08.055.

National Institutes of Mental Health. "Suicide." Accessed July 19, 2025. https://www.nimh.nih.gov/health/statistics/suicide#:~:text=100%2C000%20in%202020.-,The%20total%20age%2Dadjusted%20suicide%20rate%20in%20the%20United%20States,females%20(5.7%20per%20100%2C000).

Usall, Judith, Alejandra Pinto-Meza, Anna Fernández, Ron de Graaf, Koen Demyttenaere, Jordi Alonso, Giovanni de Girolamo, Jean Pierre Lepine, Viviane Kovess, and Josep Maria Haro. "Suicide Ideation Across Reproductive Life Cycle of Women Results from a European Epidemiological Study." *Journal of Affective Disorders* 116, no. 1 (2009): 144–47. https://doi.org/10.1016/j.jad.2008.12.006.

Zhou, Yulan, Yan Zhao, and Chunhong Chen. "Effects of Mindfulness-Based Stress Reduction on Anxiety, Depression and Sleep Quality of Women in Perimenopause Period." *International Journal of Nursing Sciences* 6, no. 2 (2019): 174–79. https://doi.org/10.1016/j.ijnss.2019.03.009.

CHAPTER 6

Paraiso, Marie Fidela R., Cecile A. Ferrando, Eric R. Sokol, Charles R. Rardin, Catherine A. Matthews, Mickey M. Karram, and Cheryl B. Iglesia. "A Randomized Clinical Trial Comparing Vaginal Laser Therapy to Vaginal Estrogen Therapy in Women with Genitourinary Syndrome of Menopause: The VeLVET Trial." *Menopause* 27, no. 1 (2020): 50–56. https://doi.org/10.1097/GME.0000000000001416.

CHAPTER 7

Islam, Rakibul M., Robin J. Bell, Sally Green, Matthew J. Page, and Susan R. Davis. "Safety and Efficacy of Testosterone for Women: A Systematic Review and Meta-Analysis of Randomised Controlled Trial Data." *The Lancet Diabetes & Endocrinology* 7, no. 10 (2019): 754–66. https://doi.org/10.1016/S2213-8587(19)30189-5.

Jiang, Xuezhi, Anna Bossert, K. Nathan Parthasarathy, Kristine Leaman, Shahab S. Minassian, Peter F. Schnatz, and Mark B. Woodland. "Safety Assessment of Compounded Non-FDA-Approved Hormonal Therapy Versus FDA-Approved Hormonal Therapy in Treating Postmenopausal Women." *Menopause* 28, no. 8 (2021): 867–74. https://doi.org/10.1097/GME.0000000000001782.

Morton, Heather, and Boris B. Gorzalka. "Role of Partner Novelty in Sexual Functioning: A Review." *Journal of Sex and Marital Therapy* 41, no. 6 (2015): 593–609. https://doi.org/10.1080/0092623X.2014.958788.

Shifren, Jan L., Brigitta U. Monz, Patricia A. Russo, Anthony Segreti, and Catherine B. Johannes. "Sexual Problems and Distress in United States Women: Prevalence and Correlates." *Obstetrics and Gynecology* 112, no. 5 (2008): 970–78. https://doi.org/10.1097/AOG.0b013e3181898cdb.

Guthrie, J. R., L. Dennerstein, J. R. Taffe, P. Lehert, and H. G. Burger. "The Menopausal Transition: A 9-Year Prospective Population-Based Study. The Melbourne Women's Midlife Health Project." *Climacteric: The Journal of the International Menopause Society* 7, no. 4 (2004): 375–89. https://doi.org/10.1080/13697130400012163.

Wilcox, A. J., Donna Day Baird, David B. Dunson, D. Robert McConnaughey, James S. Kesner, and Clarice R. Weinberg. "On the Frequency of Intercourse Around Ovulation: Evidence for Biological Influences." *Human Reproduction* 19, no. 7 (2004): 1539–43. https://doi.org/10.1093/humrep/deh305.

CHAPTER 8

Coleman, Carver J., Daniel J. McDonough, Zachary C. Pope, and C. Arden Pope. "Dose-Response Association of Aerobic and Muscle-Strengthening Physical Activity with Mortality: A National Cohort Study of 416,420 US Adults." *British Journal of Sports Medicine* 56, no. 21 (2022): 1218–23. https://doi.org/10.1136/bjsports-2022-105519.

Gordon, Brett R., Cillian P. McDowell, Mats Hallgren, Jacob D. Meyer, Mark Lyons, and Matthew P. Herring. "Association of Efficacy of Resistance Exercise Training with Depressive Symptoms: Meta-Analysis and Meta-Regression Analysis of Randomized Clinical Trials." *JAMA Psychiatry* 75, no. 6 (2018): 566–76. https://doi.org/10.1001/jamapsychiatry.2018.0572.

Markwald, Rachel R., Edward L. Melanson, Mark R. Smith, Janine Higgins, Leigh Perreault, Robert H. Eckel, and Kenneth P. Wright. "Impact of Insufficient Sleep on Total Daily Energy Expenditure, Food Intake, and Weight Gain." *Proceedings of the National Academy of Sciences* 110, no. 14 (2013): 5695–700. https://doi.org/10.1073/pnas.1216951110.

Paddon-Jones, Douglas, Eric Westman, Richard D. Mattes, Robert R. Wolfe, Arne Astrup, and Margriet Westerterp-Plantenga. "Protein, Weight Management, and Satiety." *American Journal of Clinical Nutrition* 87, no. 5 (2008): 1558S–61S. https://doi.org/10.1093/ajcn/87.5.1558S.

Patel, Sanjay R., Atul Malhotra, David P. White, Daniel J. Gottlieb, and Frank B. Hu. "Association Between Reduced Sleep and Weight Gain in Women." *American Journal of Epidemiology* 164, no. 10 (2006): 947–54. https://doi.org/10.1093/aje/kwj280.

Poehlman, E. T. "Effects of Resistance Training and Endurance Training on Insulin Sensitivity in Nonobese, Young Women: A Controlled Randomized Trial." *Journal of Clinical Endocrinology and Metabolism* 85, no. 7 (2000): 2463–68. https://doi.org/10.1210/jc.85.7.2463.

Raubenheimer, David, and Stephen J. Simpson. "Protein Leverage: Theoretical Foundations and Ten Points of Clarification." *Obesity* 27, no. 8 (2019): 1225–38. https://doi.org/10.1002/oby.22531.

Simpson, Stephen J., David Raubenheimer, Kirsten I. Black, and Arthur D.

Conigrave. "Weight Gain During the Menopause Transition: Evidence for a Mechanism Dependent on Protein Leverage." *BJOG: An International Journal of Obstetrics & Gynaecology* 130, no. 1 (2023): 4–10. https://doi.org /10.1111/1471-0528.17290.

Smith, Carly, and Stacy Sims. "Strength Training During Perimenopause." *Stanford Lifestyle Medicine.* Last updated July 11, 2023. https://longevity .stanford.edu/lifestyle/2023/07/11/strength-training-during-perimenopause/.

Srikanthan, Preethi, Tamara B. Horwich, Marcella Calfon Press, Jeff Gornbein, and Karol E. Watson. "Sex Differences in the Association of Body Composition and Cardiovascular Mortality." *Journal of the American Heart Association* 10, no. 5 (2021). https://doi.org/10.1161/JAHA.120.017511.

CHAPTER 9

Maki, P. M., and N. G. Jaff. "Brain Fog in Menopause: A Health-Care Professional's Guide for Decision-Making and Counseling on Cognition." *Climacteric: The Journal of the International Menopause Society* 25, no. 6 (2022): 570–78. https://doi.org/10.1080/13697137.2022.2122792.

Mosconi, Lisa, Matilde Nerattini, Dawn C. Matthews, Steven Jett, Caroline Andy, Schantel Williams, Camila Boneu Yepez, et al. "In Vivo Brain Estrogen Receptor Density by Neuroendocrine Aging and Relationships with Cognition and Symptomatology." *Scientific Reports* 14, no. 1 (2024). https://doi.org/10.1038/s41598-024-62820-7.

Weber, M. T., L. H. Rubin, R. Schroeder, T. Steffenella, and P. M. Maki. "Cognitive Profiles in Perimenopause: Hormonal and Menopausal Symptom Correlates." *Climacteric: The Journal of the International Menopause Society* 24, no. 4 (2021): 401–7. https://doi.org/10.1080/13697137.2021.1892626.

CHAPTER 10

Burns, Laura J., Brianna De Souza, Elizabeth Flynn, Dina Hagigeorges, and Maryanne M. Senna. "Spironolactone for Treatment of Female Pattern Hair Loss." *Journal of the American Academy of Dermatology* 83, no. 1 (2020): 276–78. https://doi.org/10.1016/j.jaad.2020.03.087.

Draelos, Zoe. "A Clinical Study to Assess the Facial Anti-Aging Efficacy of Topical Estriol and Estradiol." June 30, 2024. https://assets.ctfassets.net /md0kv0ejg0xf/4gaULAkbHbgNZtNMOgg1PI/91329de08abacf438fb83d 99e756ee99/Alloy_M4_Report_063024.pdf.

Pivazyan, Laura, Julietta Avetisyan, Maria Loshkareva, and Amina

Abdurakhmanova. "Skin Rejuvenation in Women Using Menopausal Hormone Therapy: A Systematic Review and Meta-Analysis." *Journal of Menopausal Medicine* 29, no. 3 (2023): 97.

Skin Cancer Foundation. "Melanoma Warning Signs." Accessed July 28, 2025. https://www.skincancer.org/skin-cancer-information/melanoma/melanoma -warning-signs-and-images/.

CHAPTER 11

Bansal, Ramandeep, and Neelam Aggarwal. "Menopausal Hot Flashes: A Concise Review." *Journal of Mid-Life Health* 10, no. 1 (2019): 6–13. https://doi.org/10.4103/jmh.JMH_7_19.

Halseth, Regine, Charlotte Loppie, and Nicole Robinson. *Menopause and Indigenous Women in Canada: The State of Current Research.* National Collaborating Centre for Aboriginal Health, 2018.

Hunter, M. S. "Cognitive Behavioral Therapy for Menopausal Symptoms." *Climacteric: The Journal of the International Menopause Society* 24, no. 1 (2021): 51–56. https://doi.org/10.1080/13697137.2020.1777965.

MacLennan, Alastair H., Jessica L. Broadbent, Sue Lester, and Vivienne Moore. "Oral Oestrogen and Combined Oestrogen/Progestogen Therapy versus Placebo for Hot Flushes." *Cochrane Database of Systematic Reviews* 2009, no. 1 (2004). https://doi.org/10.1002/14651858.CD002978 .pub2.

Menopause Society. "Clinical Hypnosis vs. Cognitive Behavioral Therapy: What's Better for Managing Hot Flashes?" Press release, September 10, 2024. https://menopause.org/wp-content/uploads/press-release/Hypnosis-and -CBT-for-Hot-Flashes.pdf.

Voedisch, Amy J., Rebecca Dunsmoor-Su, and Jennifer Kasirsky. "Menopause: A Global Perspective and Clinical Guide for Practice." *Clinical Obstetrics and Gynecology* 64, no. 3 (2021): 528–54. https://doi.org/10.1097/GRF .0000000000000639.

CHAPTER 12

Blümel, J. E, Camil Castelo-Branco, Luis Binfa, Raul Aparicio, and Luis Mamani. "A Scheme of Combined Oral Contraceptives for Women More Than 40 Years Old." *Menopause* 8, no. 4 (2001): 286–89. https://doi.org/10 .1097/00042192-200107000-00011.

Centers for Disease Control. "Updated Methodology to Estimate Overall and Unintended Pregnancy Rates in the United States." *Vital and Health Statistics* 2, no. 201 (April 2023): 14–16.

Chandra A., C. E. Copen, and E. H. Stephen. "Infertility and Impaired Fecundity in the United States, 1982–2010: Data from the National Survey of Family Growth." *National Health Statistics Reports* 67 (2013):1–18.

Dittrick Medical History Center. "Intrauterine Device (IUD)." Case Western University College of Arts and Sciences. Accessed December 24, 2024. https://artsci.case.edu/dittrick/online-exhibits/history-of-birth-control /contraception-in-america-1950-present-day/intrauterine-device-iud/.

Grandi, Giovanni, Pierluigi Di Vinci, Alice Sgandurra, Lia Feliciello, Francesca Monari, and Fabio Facchinetti. "Contraception During Perimenopause: Practical Guidance." *International Journal of Women's Health* 14 (2022): 913–29. https://doi.org/10.2147/IJWH.S288070.

Pernambuco-Holsten, Christina. "Birth Control and Cancer Risk: 6 Things You Should Know." Memorial Sloan Kettering Cancer Center. Last updated September 25, 2018. https://www.mskcc.org/news/birth-control-and -cancer-risk.

Planned Parenthood. "A History of Birth Control Methods." January 2012. https://www.plannedparenthood.org/files/2613/9611/6275/History_of _BC_Methods.pdf.

Planned Parenthood. "The Birth Control Pill: A History." Last updated June 2015. https://www.plannedparenthood.org/files/1514/3518/7100/Pill _History_FactSheet.pdf.

CHAPTER 13

Baik, Seo H., Fitsum Baye, and Clement J. McDonald. "Use of Menopausal Hormone Therapy Beyond Age 65 Years and Its Effects on Women's Health Outcomes by Types, Routes, and Doses." *Menopause* 31, no. 5 (2024): 363–71. https://doi.org/10.1097/GME.0000000000002335.

Cagnacci, A., and M. Venier. "The Controversial History of Hormone Replacement Therapy." *Medicina* 5, no. 9 (September 18, 2019): 602. https://doi.org/10.3390/medicina55090602.

Kohn, G. E., K. M. Rodriguez, J. Hotaling, and A. W. Pastuszak. "The History of Estrogen Therapy." *Sexual Medicine Reviews* 7, no. 3 (July 2019): 416–21. https://doi.org/10.1016/j.sxmr.2019.03.006.

Krauthammer, Charles. "When Modern Medicine Fails." *Washington Post*, July 12, 2002.

Mauvais-Jarvis, Franck, JoAnn E. Manson, John C. Stevenson, and Vivian A. Fonseca. "Menopausal Hormone Therapy and Type 2 Diabetes Prevention: Evidence, Mechanisms, and Clinical Implications." *Endocrine Reviews* 38, no. 3 (2017): 173–88. https://doi.org/10.1210/er.2016-1146.

Menopause Society. "Hormone Therapy." Accessed July 28, 2025. https:// menopause.org/patient-education/menopause-topics/hormone-therapy.

CHAPTER 14

Kim, Da Seul, Na Yeon Kim, Doug Hyun Han, Hee Jun Kim, Eun Seung Yu, and Sun Mi Kim. "Efficacy of Cognitive Behavioral Therapy for Menopausal Symptoms and Quality of Life in Korean Perimenopausal Women: A Pilot Randomized Controlled Trial." *Maturitas* 189 (2024). https://doi.org/10 .1016/j.maturitas.2024.108103.

Radzinsky, V. E., Y. Uspenskaya, L. P. Shulman, and I. V. Kuznetsova. "Succinate-Based Dietary Supplement for Menopausal Symptoms: A Pooled Analysis of Two Identical Randomized, Double-Blind, Placebo-Controlled Clinical Trials." *Obstetrics and Gynecology International* 2019 (2019): 1–9.

Shan, Dan, Li Zou, Xijiao Liu, Yongchun Shen, Yitong Cai, and Jing Zhang. "Efficacy and Safety of Gabapentin and Pregabalin in Patients with Vasomotor Symptoms: A Systematic Review and Meta-Analysis." *American Journal of Obstetrics and Gynecology* 222, no. 6 (2020): 564–79.e12. https:// doi.org/10.1016/j.ajog.2019.12.011.

CHAPTER 15

American Heart Association. "American Heart Association Recommendations for Physical Activity in Adults and Kids." Accessed July 31, 2025. https:// www.heart.org/en/healthy-living/fitness/fitness-basics/aha-recs-for-physical -activity-in-adults#:~:text=Get%20at%20least%20150%20minutes,and%20 intensity%20gradually%20over%20time.

Andersson, Tobias, Jonatan Nåtman, Georgios Mourtzinis, Johan-Emil Bager, Kristina Bengtsson Boström, Stefan Franzén, and Per Hjerpe. "The Effect of Statins on Mortality and Cardiovascular Disease in Primary Care Hypertensive Patients Without Other Cardiovascular Disease or Diabetes." *European Journal of Preventive Cardiology* 30, no. 17 (2023): 1883–94. https://doi.org/10.1093/eurjpc/zwad212.

Centers for Disease Control. "Heart Disease Risk Factors." Accessed July 31, 2025. https://www.cdc.gov/heart-disease/risk-factors/index.html.

Derby, C. A., S. L. Crawford, R. C. Pasternak, M. Sowers, B. Sternfeld, and
K. A. Matthews. "Lipid Changes During the Menopause Transition in
Relation to Age and Weight: The Study of Women's Health Across the
Nation." *American Journal of Epidemiology* 169, no. 11 (2009): 1352–61.
https://doi.org/10.1093/aje/kwp043.

Jeffers, Abra M., Stanton Glantz, Amy L. Byers, and Salomeh Keyhani.
"Association of Cannabis Use with Cardiovascular Outcomes Among US
Adults." *Journal of the American Heart Association* 13, no. 5 (2024). https://
doi.org/10.1161/JAHA.123.030178.

Khamis, Ramzi Y., Tareq Ammari, and Ghada W. Mikhail. "Gender Differences
in Coronary Heart Disease." *Heart* (British Cardiac Society) 102, no. 14
(2016): 1142–49. https://doi.org/10.1136/heartjnl-2014-306463.

Merschel, Michael. "How Much Harm Can a Little Excess Salt Do? Plenty."
American Heart Association. Last updated May 26, 2021. https://www.heart
.org/en/news/2021/05/26/how-much-harm-can-a-little-excess-salt-do-plenty.

Newsom, Rob. "Sleep Apnea and Heart Disease." Sleep Foundation. Last
updated July 15, 2025. https://www.sleepfoundation.org/sleep-apnea/sleep
-apnea-linked-heart-disease.

Shan, Zhilei, Yanping Li, Megu Y. Baden, Shilpa N. Bhupathiraju, Dong
D. Wang, Qi Sun, Kathryn M. Rexrode, et al. "Association Between
Healthy Eating Patterns and Risk of Cardiovascular Disease." *JAMA
Internal Medicine* 180, no. 8 (2020): 1090–1100. https://doi.org/10.1001
/jamainternmed.2020.2176.

University of Michigan News. "Weight Training Can Improve Heart Disease
Risk Factors in Just 30 Minutes a Week." Accessed July 31, 2025. https://
news.umich.edu/weight-training-can-improve-heart-disease-risk-factors
-in-just-30-minutes-a-week/#:~:text=The%20list%20of%20people%20
for,doctor%20before%20beginning%20a%20program.

CHAPTER 16

Anderson, Heather. "BRCA and Your Cancer Risk: What You Need to Know."
M.D. Anderson Cancer Center. Last updated November 2018. https://www
.mdanderson.org/publications/focused-on-health/brca-and-your-cancer
-risk--what-you-need-to-know.h20-1592202.html.

Centers for Disease Control and Prevention. "People at Increased Risk for
BRCA Gene Mutation." Last updated September 3, 2024. https://www.cdc
.gov/breast-ovarian-cancer-hereditary/risk-factors/index.html.

Hamajima, N., K. Hirose, K. Tajima, T. Rohan, E. E. Calle, C. W. Heath, R. J. Coates, et al. "Alcohol, Tobacco and Breast Cancer—Collaborative Reanalysis of Individual Data from 53 Epidemiological Studies, Including 58,515 Women with Breast Cancer and 95,067 Women Without the Disease." *British Journal of Cancer* 87, no. 11 (2002): 1234–45. https://doi.org/10.1038/sj.bjc.6600596.

Lo, Jamie J., Yong-Moon Mark Park, Rashmi Sinha, and Dale P. Sandler. "Association Between Meat Consumption and Risk of Breast Cancer: Findings from the Sister Study." *International Journal of Cancer* 146, no. 8 (2020): 2156–65. https://doi.org/10.1002/ijc.32547.

Munir, Javeria, Yashmin Nisha, Nayaar Islam, Mary Beth Bissell, Betty Anne Schwarz, Erin Cordeiro, and Jean M. Seely. "Impact of Method of Detection of Breast Cancer on Clinical Outcomes in Individuals Aged 40 Years or Older." *Radiology: Imaging Cancer* 7, no. 3 (2025). https://doi.org/10.1148/rycan.240046.

Mutch, David. "Why Annual Pap Smears Are History—But Routine Ob-Gyn Visits Are Not." American College of Obstetricians and Gynecologists. Accessed August 6, 2025. https://www.acog.org/womens-health/experts-and-stories/the-latest/why-annual-pap-smears-are-history-but-routine-ob-gyn-visits-are-not.

National Cancer Institute. "BRCA Gene Changes: Cancer Risk and Genetic Testing." Accessed July 31, 2025. https://www.cancer.gov/about-cancer/causes-prevention/genetics/brca-fact-sheet.

National Cancer Institute. "Browse the SEER Cancer Statistics Review (CSR) 1975–2017." Accessed February 8, 2025. https://seer.cancer.gov/archive/csr/1975_2017/browse_csr.php?sectionSEL=4&pageSEL=sect_04_table.17.

National Cancer Institute. "Obesity and Cancer." Accessed July 31, 2025. https://www.cancer.gov/about-cancer/causes-prevention/risk/obesity/obesity-fact-sheet.

Richman, Ilana B., Jessica B. Long, Pamela R. Soulos, Shi-Yi Wang, and Cary P. Gross. "Estimating Breast Cancer Overdiagnosis After Screening Mammography Among Older Women in the United States." *Annals of Internal Medicine* 176, no. 9 (2023): 1172–80. https://doi.org/10.7326/M23-0133.

Susan G. Komen. "Breast Cancer Risk Factors: Birth Control Pills and Other Hormonal Birth Control." Accessed July 31, 2025. https://www.komen.org/breast-cancer/risk-factor/birth-control-pills/.

Susan G. Komen. "Research Table: Smoking and Breast Cancer Risk." Accessed July 31, 2025. https://www.komen.org/breast-cancer/facts-statistics /research-studies/topics/smoking-and-breast-cancer-risk/.

Wisdom. "Study Overview." Accessed August 6, 2025. https://www .thewisdomstudy.org/learn-more/#study-overview.

CHAPTER 17

Bone Health and Osteoporosis Foundation. "What Women Need to Know." Accessed August 9, 2025. https://www.bonehealthandosteoporosis.org /preventing-fractures/general-facts/what-women-need-to-know/.

Cawthon, Peggy M. "Gender Differences in Osteoporosis and Fractures." *Clinical Orthopaedics and Related Research* 469, no. 7 (2011): 1900–1905. https://doi.org/10.1007/s11999-011-1780-7.

Chin, K. Y. "The Relationship Between Follicle-Stimulating Hormone and Bone Health: Alternative Explanation for Bone Loss Beyond Oestrogen?" *International Journal of Medical Sciences* 15, no. 12 (September 7, 2018): 1373–83. https://doi.org/10.7150/ijms.26571.

Ciosek, Żaneta, Karolina Kot, Danuta Kosik-Bogacka, Natalia Łanocha-Arendarczyk, and Iwona Rotter. "The Effects of Calcium, Magnesium, Phosphorus, Fluoride, and Lead on Bone Tissue." *Biomolecules* 11, no. 4 (2021). https://doi.org/10.3390/biom11040506.

Fernández-Rodríguez, Rubén, Celia Alvarez-Bueno, Sara Reina-Gutiérrez, Ana Torres-Costoso, Sergio Nuñez de Arenas-Arroyo, and Vicente Martínez-Vizcaíno. "Effectiveness of Pilates and Yoga to Improve Bone Density in Adult Women: A Systematic Review and Meta-Analysis." *PLoS One* 16, no. 5 (2021). https://doi.org/10.1371/journal.pone.025139.

Godos, Justyna, Francesca Giampieri, Emanuele Chisari, Agnieszka Micek, Nadia Paladino, Tamara Y. Forbes-Hernández, José L. Quiles, et al. "Alcohol Consumption, Bone Mineral Density, and Risk of Osteoporotic Fractures: A Dose-Response Meta-Analysis." *International Journal of Environmental Research and Public Health* 19, no. 3 (2022). https://doi.org/10.3390 /ijerph19031515.

International Osteoporosis Foundation. "Risk Factors." Accessed August 11, 2025. https://www.osteoporosis.foundation/patients/about-osteoporosis /risk-factors.

Katsoulis, M., V. Benetou, T. Karapetyan, D. Feskanich, F. Grodstein, U. Pettersson-Kymmer, S. Eriksson, et al. "Excess Mortality After Hip Fracture in Elderly Persons from Europe and the USA: The CHANCES Project." *Journal of Internal Medicine* 281, no. 3 (2017): 300–310. https://doi.org/10.1111/joim.12586.

Maurel, D. B., N. Boisseau, C. L. Benhamou, and C. Jaffre. "Alcohol and Bone: Review of Dose Effects and Mechanisms." *Osteoporosis International* 23, no. 1 (2012): 1–16. https://doi.org/10.1007/s00198-011-1787-7.

Medical News Today. "Do Only Women Develop Osteoporosis?" Accessed August 9, 2025. https://www.medicalnewstoday.com/articles/only-women-develop-osteoporosis.

Index

ablation, 51, 97

acne, 143, 147, 151, 155, 172, 179, 184

acupuncture, 165–66

Addyi, 113

adenomyosis, 45, 46

adrenal glands, 28, 31, 38

aging, 22–24

Aldactone, 150

Alzheimer's disease, 23

Amberen, 201

Ambien, 66

American Association of Sexuality Educators, Counselors and Therapists (AASECT), 109

ammonium succinate, 201

AndroFem, 110

andropause, 19

anger, 1, 27, 30, 72, 73, 75, 82

anti-anxiety medications, 48, 55, 87

anticholinergics, 66

antidepressants, 72, 75, 85, 86–88, 106, 131, 168, 236

anxiety, 14, 72, 75, 76–77; anti-anxiety medications, 48, 55, 87; contraception and, 175; general anxiety disorder (GAD), 76; menopausal hormone therapy and, 139, 140; progesterone and, 30, 37; sleep and, 56–57, 58, 59–60, 68; treatments for, 83, 85, 86–87, 202–3, 204

Asian women, 25, 158, 233

attention deficit hyperactivity disorder (ADHD), 137–38, 141

autoimmune disorders, 17, 93, 94, 96, 97, 98–99, 145, 236

BedJet, 164

Benadryl, 66

biopsies: breast, 228; uterine, 47–48

biotin (vitamin B7), 149

birth control pills, 170–71, 174, 175, 176–82, 199; acne and, 151; breast cancer and, 223; for erratic and heavy bleeding, 49, 50; esterol in, 29; hair growth and, 150–51; for mood issues, 85–86; for polycystic ovary syndrome, 16; for sleep issues, 67–68

bisphenol A (BPA), 21

black cohosh, 164–65

Black women, 25, 45, 47, 80, 158, 219–20, 233

bladder issues and infections, 94–95, 99–100. *See also* incontinence, urinary

bleeding. *See* periods, erratic

bone density, 232–42; aging and, 234–37; alcohol and, 237; estrogen and, 233, 235, 237, 240; medications and, 236, 241–42; menopausal hormone therapy and, 190–91, 193, 232, 234, 241; nutrition and, 238–40; osteoporosis, 191, 193, 232–33, 235, 236, 237, 238, 239–41; physical activity and, 240–41; risk reduction, 237–42

bone density scans, 233–34

brain fog, 133–42; attention deficit hyperactivity disorder and, 137–38, 141; causes of, 134–38; hot flashes and,

brain fog (*continued*)
138, 139–40; menopausal hormone therapy for, 139–40; sleep and, 134, 138, 139–40; symptoms of, 134–35; treatments for, 138–42
breast cancer, 219–31; aging and risk of, 220–23; alcohol and, 222; BRCA mutations and, 221, 226; contraception and, 183–84, 223–24; contraindicated screenings for, 229–30; hormones and, 223–24; mammograms and other screenings, 225–40, 247; menopausal hormone therapy and, 224; nutrition and, 222–23; obesity and, 223; risk management, 225–31; treatments for, 228–29
Broderick, Meredith, 60, 61

calcium, 214, 236, 238, 239
cancer screenings, 230–31
cannabis and cannabidiol products, 67, 140, 213
cardiovascular health, 209–18; aging and, 210–11; alcohol and, 213; blood pressure and, 216; diabetes and, 215; estrogen and, 209, 211, 218; heart attacks, 163, 177, 188–89, 211–12, 213, 214, 217; inflammation and, 211, 214, 217; lipid and blood sugar testing, 216–17; menopausal hormone therapy and, 211, 217–18; nutrition and, 213–14; obesity and, 216; physical activity and, 214–15; risk reduction, 212–15; sleep apnea and, 216; smoking and, 213
Chilipad, 69, 164, 200
clinical hypnosis, 166, 199, 202–3
clitoris, 91, 111
cognitive behavioral therapy (CBT), 84–85, 124, 140, 166, 202–3
cognitive behavioral therapy for insomnia (CBT-I), 64–66, 85
contraception, 171–86; breast cancer and, 183, 184; combined hormonal contraception, 174–75; Dalkon Shield, 183; Depo-Provera, 185–86, 224; estrogen and, 173, 174, 175–82, 184–85, 186; how it helps

perimenopausal symptoms, 174–76; injections and implants, 185–86; intrauterine devices (IUDs), 49, 50, 171–72, 182–85, 204, 224; Nexplanon, 186; progesterone and, 174, 178; progestin-only contraception, 176, 180–81, 185, 196, 198. *See also* birth control pills
cortisol, 58, 77, 122
COVID-19 pandemic, 72, 227–28

Darwinism, 33, 162
Davis, Susan R., 110
dementia: aging and, 23; anticholinergics and, 66; brain fog versus, 134, 142; menopausal hormone therapy and, 188, 190, 197
depression, 72, 74–75, 77–80; antidepressants, 72, 75, 85, 86–88, 106, 131, 168, 236; brain fog and, 138; contraception and, 175; major depressive disorder, 72, 78; menopausal hormone therapy and, 139, 140; postpartum depression (PPD), 78, 85; progesterone and, 30, 37, 78; signs of, 80; sleep and, 56; treatments for, 83, 85, 86, 88, 126, 202, 205
Desyrel, 66
diabetes, 118, 126, 128, 130, 191, 215–17, 223
diphenhydramine, 66
divorce, 81–82, 108
Dominus, Susan, 2
dopamine, 30, 67, 75, 131, 137–38

early menopause, 17, 25
Elagolix, 49–50
elinzanetant, 167
endocrine disruptors, 20–21
endometriosis, 15, 52–53, 183
estradiol, 29; combined with IUDs, 183, 184–85; ethinyl estradiol, 178, 179, 180–81; in face creams, 151, 152; in menopausal hormone therapy, 193–94, 195–98
estrogen, 28–29; ADHD and, 137–38; bone density and, 233, 235, 237, 240; brain fog and, 134–37, 139, 141;

cardiovascular health and, 209, 211, 218; contraception and, 173, 174, 175–82, 184–85, 186; estetrol, 29; estriol, 29, 151, 152; estrone, 29, 119; in face creams, 152–53; hair symptoms and, 145, 146; insulin resistance and, 126; libido and, 104, 106, 111, 112–13; in menopausal hormone therapy, 31, 189–93, 194–97, 198, 218; mood and, 74–75, 77; patch delivery, 185, 186, 204; skin symptoms and, 147, 151–53; sleep and, 59; tamoxifen and, 229; types of, 29; vaginal estrogen, 95, 96, 98, 99, 100, 152–53; vaginal symptoms and, 90, 91, 93, 95–96, 98–100; weight gain and, 118–19, 123, 126. *See also* estradiol
eszopiclone, 66
exercise. *See* physical activity and exercise

fertilization, 15, 28–29, 33–35, 37, 43, 73, 161, 174
fezolinetant, 167, 205
fibroids, 25, 45–46, 47, 48, 49, 51
fight-or-flight, 77, 122, 203
final menstrual period (FMP), 4, 17, 79–80, 162, 182, 189, 248
flibanserin, 113
follicle-stimulating hormone (FSH), 28, 34–36, 37–38, 73, 75, 161, 174, 237
Fortamet, 131
Fuller, Ashley, 108

gabapentin, 204–5
Gamma-aminobutyric acid (GABA), 30, 67, 75, 204–5
general anxiety disorder (GAD), 76. *See also* anxiety
genitourinary syndrome of menopause (GSM), 106
ghrelin, 119, 120
GLP-1 medications, 129–31
Glumetza, 131
gonadotropin-releasing hormone (GnRH), 34, 49–50, 161–62
grandmother hypothesis, 18
gray divorce, 81–82, 108

hair symptoms, 144–47; alopecia, 145; estrogen and, 145, 146; female-pattern baldness, 144, 149, 150; hair loss, 144–46; menopausal hormone therapy and, 150; new hair growth, 146–47; telogen effluvium, 145–46; treatments for, 149–51
healthcare providers, choosing, 243–52; Menopause Society Certified Practitioners, 6, 246; nurse practitioners (NPs), 246; Perimenopause Appointment Checklist, 250–51, 252; perimenopause/menopause specialists, 246
health disparities, 25–26, 219–20
heart palpitations, 76–77, 211
Hispanic women, 25, 158, 220
hormone replacement therapy (HRT). *See* menopausal hormone therapy
hormone testing, 12–13
hot flashes and night sweats, 157–68; brain fog and, 138, 139–40; causes of, 161–64; Chilipad for, 69, 164, 200; estrogen and, 160, 161, 163, 164, 165, 166–67; heart attacks versus, 211–12; night sweats, 62–63, 68, 69, 140, 159, 162, 164, 167, 189; persistent hot flashes, 163–64; phthalates and, 21; treatments for, 164–68
Hot Flash Related Daily Interference Scale, 65
hypnotherapy, 166, 199, 202–3
hypothalamus, 34, 161–62
hysterectomy, 25, 48, 51–52, 229, 250
hysteria, 1–2
hysteroscopy, 48, 50–51

ibuprofen, 49
incontinence, urinary, 94, 98–100, 123, 159–60, 167, 193, 203, 205
inflammation, 53, 189, 211, 214, 217, 220, 236
intrauterine devices (IUDs), 49, 50, 171–72, 182–85, 204, 224
iron: dietary and supplementary, 53–54; low iron levels, 145
irritability, 3, 24, 30, 56, 72, 75, 105, 201

Jaff, Nicole, 136–37, 138

Kabat-Zinn, Jon, 83
Kasianchu, Stasi, 125–26, 129
Kegel exercises, 99
KNDy neuron, 161–62, 167
Krejci, Sonja M., 153, 156

layering treatments, 87, 204–5
leptin, 119, 120, 223
leuprolide, 49
libido, 32, 87, 101–14; arousal disorders, 106–7; genitourinary syndrome of menopause (GSM), 106; hot flashes and, 105; mood swings and, 105; persistent genital arousal disorder (PGAD), 106; progesterone and, 104, 106, 111, 112–13; sleep and, 105; stress and, 105; testosterone and, 104, 109–12, 113; treatments for, 107–13
lichen sclerosus, 93, 94, 96, 97, 98–99
Lunesta, 66
Lupron, 49
luteinizing hormone (LH), 34–35, 174
Lysteda, 49, 50

Maki, Pauline, 136–37, 138
male menopause, 19
marijuana and cannabis, 67, 140, 213
medical school, 4
meditation, 83, 140–41, 166
melatonin, 58, 63, 67
menopausal hormone therapy (MHT), 187–98; benefits of, 190–91; bone density and, 190–91, 193, 232, 234, 241; brain fog and, 139–40; breast cancer and, 191–92, 197, 198, 224; cardiovascular health and, 211, 217–18; contraindications for, 192; dementia and, 188, 190, 197; ending treatment, 197–98; estradiol in, 193–98; estrogen in, 31, 189–93, 194–97, 198, 218; hair symptoms and, 150; hormone sources for, 194–95; mood and, 85, 86–87, 139, 140; options for, 193–97; progesterone, 187, 191–92, 193–94, 196–97; progesterone in, 68, 166, 187, 191–92, 193–94, 196–97;

risks and side effects of, 190, 191–92; sleep and, 68–69; transdermal delivery systems, 194; vaginal ring, 195–96; weight gain and, 129–30; window of opportunity to begin treatment, 189
menopause: definition of, 2, 15; in nonhuman animals, 18–19; perimenopause to, 37–38; perimenopause versus, 2, 15
Menopause Research and Equity Act, 19–20
Menopause Society, 165, 166, 202, 203, 246
Menopause Society Certified Practitioner (MSCP), 6, 246
menstruation. *See* periods, erratic; premenstrual syndrome; puberty
mental health. *See* mood and mental health
metformin, 16, 131
Millheiser, Leah, 106
minoxidil, 149–50
Mintz, Laurie B., 108
mood and mental health, 71–88; divorce and, 81–82; menopausal hormone therapy for, 85, 86–87; post-traumatic stress disorder (PTSD), 77, 204; progesterone and, 30, 37, 74–75, 78; treatments for, 80–81, 83–88. *See also* anxiety; depression
Mosconi, Lisa, 136
movement. *See* physical activity and exercise
muscle mass, loss of, 32, 62, 235
myomectomy, 51

naltrexone, 131
National Health and Nutrition Examination Survey (NHANES), 20–21
National Institutes of Health (NIH), 19–20
New Relationship Energy, 105
night sweats. *See* hot flashes and night sweats
nonhormonal prescription medications, 204–5
nonprescription medical interventions, 202–4
Nurses' Health Study, 121

obesity, 130, 192, 216, 223. *See also* weight gain
OBGYNs for a Sustainable Future, 20

oocytes, 32–33, 35–36

osteoporosis, 191, 193, 232–33, 235, 236, 237, 238, 239–41. *See also* bone density

mittelschmerz (pain or bleeding during ovulation), 41–54

palpitations, heart, 76–77, 211

panic attacks, 12, 24, 76

paroxetine, 168

pelvic floor therapy, 99–100

Penn Ovarian Aging Study, 79–80

perimenopause: definition of, 2, 12, 14–15; environmental conditions that affect, 20–21; hormonal conditions that affect, 15–18; to menopause, 37–38; menopause versus, 2, 15; in nonhuman animals, 18–19; puberty to, 35–37

periods, erratic, 41–54; endometriosis and, 52–53; evaluations and tests, 42–48; iron levels and, 53–54; reasons for, 42–45; treatments for, 48–52

persistent genital arousal disorder (PGAD), 106

PFAS (per and polyfluoroalkyl substances), 20

phentermine, 131

phthalates, 20–21

physical activity and exercise: bone density and, 240–41; brain fog and, 140; cardiovascular exercise, 128–29, 140; cardiovascular health and, 214–15; mood and, 83; strength training, 118, 121, 126–28, 131, 215, 216, 238, 241; weight gain and, 126–29

polycystic ovary syndrome (PCOS), 16–17, 147

polyps, 45, 46–47, 48, 50–51

positron emission tomography (PET) imaging, 136

post-traumatic stress disorder (PTSD), 77, 204

precancers, 30, 45, 46, 47, 123, 184, 229

premature menopause, 25, 190

Premature ovarian insufficiency (POI), 17–18

premenopause, 14, 42, 57, 61, 74, 91, 187

premenstrual dysphoric disorder (PMDD), 87–88, 175

premenstrual syndrome (PMS), 74, 78, 85, 87, 174–75

progesterone, 30–31; contraception and, 174, 178; libido and, 104, 106, 111, 112–13; luteinizing hormone and, 34–35; in menopausal hormone therapy, 68, 166, 187, 191–92, 193–94, 196–97; micronized progesterone, 67, 68, 192, 196–97; mood and, 30, 37, 74–75, 78; sleep and, 59, 62, 67–68

progestins, 31, 68, 151, 174, 176–77, 179–86, 194, 196–98

progestogens, 30–31, 68, 173, 174, 196

protein, dietary, 125–26, 238

puberty, 14, 27–28, 33, 35, 73–74

puberty, second, 27–28, 73, 147

purified cytoplasm of pollen (PCP), 201

Relugolix, 49–50

semaglutide, 130

serotonin, 75, 78, 113

sex hormone–binding globulin (SHBG), 31, 147, 151

sex therapy, 106, 109

sexual dysfunction. *See* libido

skin and nail symptoms, 147–48; acne, 143, 147, 151, 155, 172, 179, 184; dryness, 147–48; estrogen and, 147, 151–53; melanoma, 154; sensitive skin, 155; sunscreen and, 153–54, 156; treatments for, 151–56

sleep, 55–70; aging and, 22–23; anxiety and, 56–57, 58, 59–60, 68; blue light and, 63–64; brain fog and, 134, 138, 139–40; circadian rhythm and, 58, 59, 62–63, 68; cognitive behavioral therapy for insomnia (CBT-I), 64–66, 85; hot flashes and, 62–63, 68, 69–70; melatonin and, 58, 63, 67; menopausal hormone therapy and, 68–69; pharmaceuticals for, 55, 66–69; progesterone and, 59, 62, 67–68; purposes of, 56; stages of, 57–58; waking after sleep onset (WASO), 23, 60; weight gain and, 61–62, 120, 121–22

sleep apnea, 60–62, 123, 216, 251

sleep divorce, 69–70, 107

sleep hygiene tips, 63–64

Sleep in Midlife Women Study, 61

social connection, 84

soy isoflavones, 164–65
spironolactone, 150, 151
stellate ganglion block, 203–4
stress, 24, 76–77, 83–84, 88, 105, 107, 122
suicide and suicidality, 78–79, 80, 84, 87–88
sunscreen, 153–54, 156, 239
supplements and vitamins, 201–2; biotin
     (vitamin B7), 149; black cohosh,
     164–65; vitamin C, 53, 156; vitamin
     D, 238–39
surgical menopause, 15, 25
SWAN study (Study of Women's Health
     Across the Nation), 25, 58–59, 62, 163

tamoxifen, 168, 229
testosterone, 21, 31–32, 36, 118; bone
     density and, 235; hair growth and,
     146–47, 150–51; libido and, 104,
     109–12, 113; polycystic ovary
     syndrome and, 16; sleep and, 74; trans
     men and, 19; weight gain and, 118–19
testosterone pellets, 109, 111–13, 243
tirzepitide, 130
tranexamic acid, 49, 50
transgender population, 19
trazodone, 66, 68
treatments for skin symptoms, 151–56

uterine artery embolization (uterine fibroid
     embolization), 51

vaginal anatomy, 90–91
vaginal and vulvar symptoms, 89–100;
     discharge and smell, 90, 92, 93;
     dryness, 90, 91, 92–93, 95–96, 97, 105,
     152, 195; irritation, 90, 92, 93, 95, 96;

lichen sclerosus, 93, 94, 96, 97, 98–99;
     pain during intercourse, 90, 91, 93,
     96, 97, 100; pelvic floor therapy for,
     99–100; treatments for, 95–100
vaginal estrogen, 95, 96, 98, 99, 100, 152–53
vaginal hygiene, 92–93
vaginal moisturizers, 95–96
vaginal rejuvenation, 97–98, 99
van Dis, Jane, 20
VeLVET Trial, 98
Veozah, 167, 205
vitamin C, 53, 156
vitamin D, 238–39
vulvar symptoms. *See* vaginal and vulvar
     symptoms
Vyleesi (bremelanotide), 113

Wegovy, 130
weight gain, 115–32; aging and, 23, 119–20;
     medications for, 129–32; menopausal
     hormone therapy and, 129–30;
     nutrition and, 124–26, 129; physical
     activity and, 126–29; sleep and, 61–62,
     120, 121–22; subcutaneous and
     visceral fat, 117–18; treatments for,
     122–32
white women, 25, 80, 233, 240
WISDOM study, 226–27
Women's Health Initiative (WHI), 5, 188,
     190, 191, 192
Women's Midlife Health Project, 102

yeast infections, 92

Zepbound, 130
zolpidem, 66

About the Authors

Dr. Rebecca Dunsmoor-Su is a board-certified ob-gyn and certified menopause practitioner through the Menopause Society. She is the chief medical officer at Gennev, a telemedicine platform specializing in perimenopause and menopause; co–medical director at Seattle Clinical Research Center; and an associate clinical professor of obstetrics and gynecology at Washington State University. She holds a master's in clinical epidemiology from the University of Pennsylvania.

Dr. Amy Voedisch is a board-certified ob-gyn and certified menopause practitioner through the Menopause Society. She is an associate clinical professor of obstetrics and gynecology at Stanford University and board certified in complex family planning. She holds a master's in epidemiology and clinical research from Stanford University.